Childbearing
REDEEMED

Childbearing REDEEMED

*A journey
of suffering
and hope*

ANNA VROON

Childbearing Redeemed
A journey of suffering and hope
Published by Anna Vroon with Castle Publishing
New Zealand

© 2020 Anna Vroon

ISBN 978-0-473-51551-5 (Softcover)
ISBN 978-0-473-51552-2 (ePUB)
ISBN 978-0-473-51553-9 (Kindle)

Editing: Sally Webster

Production & Typesetting:
Andrew Killick
Castle Publishing Services
www.castlepublishing.co.nz

Cover illustration:
Sara Lloyd

Cover design:
Paul Smith

Unless otherwise stated, scripture quotations are from
The Holy Bible, English Standard Version®,
copyright © 2001 by Crossway Bibles,
a publishing ministry of Good News Publishers.
Used by permission. All rights reserved.

ALL RIGHTS RESERVED

No part of this publication may be reproduced,
stored in a retrieval system, or transmitted
in any form or by any means, electronic, mechanical,
photocopying, recording or otherwise,
without prior written permission from the author.

Foreword

How can you put into words what you do not understand yourself?

Anna Vroon asks this poignant question as she shares, years after the fact, the complicated emotions around her difficult pregnancies and childbirth experiences. How do you reconcile a deep and fierce mother's love with fear, anxiety, and disgust at your pregnant belly? How do you bond with your child when you are still experiencing deep trauma after an excruciatingly painful birth process? How do you live in light of the truth of God's love and His purposes for you and your children when your emotions do not match any of it?

Anna faces these questions honestly because she experienced them all personally. In recounting her own painful journey, she has given the Church a unique and invaluable resource on pregnancy, childbirth, and motherhood. She gives women permission to be honest about their own painful stories around pregnancy and childbirth, something, frankly, few resources in the Church do. And she leads those with painful stories to the foot of the cross, where they meet the suffering Saviour who is well acquainted with searing pain and grief.

If you have wrestled with pregnancy and childbirth, despaired of giving birth, or struggled to bond with a child – or if you love someone who has – Anna has written a book you need to read. Her story is compelling, and the hope she shares in the good news of Jesus will bless every reader. I can't recommend this book enough.

Wendy Alsup
Author, *Companions in Suffering:
Comfort for Times of Loss and Loneliness*

Contents

Acknowledgements	9
Preface	11
Part One: My Story	**13**
1. An Answered Prayer	15
2. A Life Drained of Colour	21
3. Haunted by Trauma	25
4. Hope of Redemption	37
5. The Emptying	43
6. The Bottom of the Pit (Where Jesus is Found)	57
Part Two: Babies and the Bible	**67**
7. The Blessing and the Curse	69
8. In Pain	73
9. You Are Not Alone	79
10. Joy	99
Epilogue	105
Endnotes	107
About the Author	110

Acknowledgements

To the friends who endured with me through my pregnancies. I am not sure I would have hung in there if I was you, but I am deeply thankful you did.

To the women who have shared your birth stories with me. Particularly the painful ones. I am sorry for your pain. But I am grateful for the companionship in suffering. Thank you.

To Wendy Alsup, for being willing to read the first draft of this book and for your encouragement and feedback. I have learned so much from you, and am humbled by your willingness to contribute to this project. Thank you.

To my friend Zack Eswine, thank you for taking the time to read my manuscript and give thoughtful feedback and sincere encouragement which helped convince me it was worth pursuing publishing.

To my friend Sara Lloyd for your artistic talents and support.

To all those who have helped in this project; the team at Castle, those who helped with editing, proof-reading, and encouraging me by your support. I don't take it for granted and am truly grateful.

To my children – Piper, Teddy, Billy, Atua, and the ones I cannot name. This book is such a small part of my parenting journey, and although the suffering is real and deep, the joy you have brought me is far greater. I am thankful for each one of you.

And lastly, to my husband. For loving me and for living with me in an understanding way because I was the weaker vessel. I love you.

Preface

Facing my third pregnancy was like equipping myself for a battle that had broken me before and would potentially do so again. I was terrified. But I wanted to equip myself for the fight as best I could. As I walked the difficult road of pregnancy, fighting for sanity and peace, I looked to the Bible for the Lord's voice in all of this. It wasn't what I was expecting, and I wouldn't say that I won the battle. But that is part of the bigger picture, and the lessons taught could not have been learned any other way. Had things been easier for me, I might never have stopped to listen to the voice of Scripture and the language of pain. Had I not failed to end strong and victorious, I would never have known the humble grace of seeing Jesus fighting on my behalf and carrying me, both of us blood-stained and broken, across the finish line. It is a different kind of victory.

I write this book with the purpose of encouraging women who suffer in childbearing. I hope that through it you will find that the Bible speaks into your circumstances with grace, hope and joy. I hope you find, as I did, that once you let go of your ideals, then your hands are free to cling to Jesus.

PART ONE

My Story

'You're afraid of it?'

It seemed such a silly question and I spoke sharply, I think, when I said, 'Of course I am – I'm terrified.'

'Why?' he asked. 'If you lose your reason you lose it into the hands of God.'

– Elizabeth Goudge [1]

CHAPTER ONE

An Answered Prayer

I always wanted to be a wife and mother. To be honest, I really thought that was what women were supposed to be. I genuinely loved children, and had worked both as a nanny and in early childhood centres before I had my own. My desire for having my own babies had waned somewhat by the time I married, and I wasn't in too much of a hurry. Life with other people's offspring had tempered my immediate desire for my own. Being married was new and fun, and we enjoyed it unhindered by children for a year. And then the prospect of being parents became more and more appealing.

It didn't happen straight away; it took nine months of hope and disappointment. It wasn't a very long time, in retrospect, but each month it grew more disappointing, and I could not have known at the time it would only take nine months.

Taking a call from a friend who had got pregnant straightaway, only hours after I had discovered that once again I wasn't, reduced me to tears. I prayed and pleaded with the Lord. I wondered why I had to take the hard road. I didn't want the hard lesson. But as I prayed and pleaded, I came to a point where I accepted that if God had chosen the hard lesson for me then I would accept it. My prayer now was that he would grant me the gift of pregnancy that he might be glorified. I thought I was just asking for a baby, but the path to his being glorified in my life through this was more painful than I could have imagined. I didn't understand that for him to be glorified, I first must be emptied of myself.

My husband Bruwer and I were elated when I found out I was pregnant. That joyful little secret that I now carried made me wonder how I could ever be unhappy again. Ironically, it was only two weeks later that I was wondering how I could ever be happy again; I felt so sick and miserable. I suffered intense and unrelenting nausea, vomiting and migraines, and I was sicker than I had ever been in my life. I was caring for pre-schoolers in our home at the time, and remember being violently sick in the toilet as I heard families arriving to drop off their children. I can remember opening the door, my eyes still watering, and trying to smile and look enthusiastic about the prospect of spending the day with their children. As soon as the children left in the late afternoon I would go back to bed and stay there until the next morning, when I would wake feeling so sick I didn't know how I was going to get through another day. I was utterly miserable. Bruwer was kind and patient, and helped in whatever way he could. He drove all over town looking for watermelon, which wasn't in season yet, just because it was all I felt like eating.

The sickness passed about halfway through my pregnancy. The simple pleasures of cooking and eating a meal were once again mine. But a different type of affliction began to emerge as the pregnancy wore on.

The first sign was at my scan. Someone had told me it would be emotional. 'Take a box of tissues,' they had said. But I lay there looking at the monitor, and I didn't feel moved. It felt surreal and horrible. There was something alive inside my body, and I didn't like it. But I was *supposed* to love it. I felt awful about it. Did I not like my baby? I didn't know my baby, so how could I like it? I hated the feeling of it moving around inside me, and hated my distended stomach. Also, I had several weeks of severe insomnia, which did nothing to help my state of mind. I was miserable but tried to hide it. The more pregnant I became, the more disgusted I felt with it. I didn't want people to see me pregnant; I wished I was living in the days when women went into confinement. I wanted to hide, only to emerge when myself again.

Around this time Bruwer and I moved to Bible College for him to pursue theological studies, with the hope of entering pastoral ministry. We had both studied at Bible College before we were married, and we enjoyed being back there, reconnecting with old friends. We moved into a tiny flat on campus, which was to be our home for the next two years. Pregnancy aside, I was very happy there.

I was pretty good at pretending things were fine regarding the pregnancy. People would comment on how special it was, and what a wonderful time it was being pregnant. I hid my distaste for it like a dirty secret. Was there something wrong with me? I could not believe I was the first women in the world to feel this way about pregnancy, yet found no one who seemed to share my experience.

I wondered if I would ever love my baby. I didn't feel connected to it. It was living inside my body, and it felt like a violation, not a bundle of joy. One night, heavily pregnant and in the bath, I watched the baby as it twisted and turned in my stomach. I remember the panic rising inside me – I just wanted to get it out. I wildly imagined tearing my stomach open to get rid of it.

I wanted it to be over and yet, how would I feel when it was born? I didn't know. I was prepared for it to take time for us to bond, not to experience an instant connection, but for love to grow over time.

The last weeks were an agony of waiting. I longed for the pregnancy to be over, for this journey of misery to end, for this being to be separated from my body. Soon I was five days overdue, and as anyone who has been overdue knows, those five days felt like an eternity, waiting for the pain to start every moment of every day.

It was a slow start when it did come. That night the contractions were strong enough to keep me awake, but they faded as the day started. I walked and walked and tried to get things moving, but it wasn't until the evening that they started back again, this time even stronger, and sleep was impossible. They were still not regular enough to warrant going to the hospital though. The midwife checked me the next day and said I was definitely in the first stage of labour and that maybe things would happen that night.

A couple of friends popped in to visit that day as I thought it would help pass the time, but I remember hiding my face behind my husband's back when the contractions came so they wouldn't see how much pain I was in. I didn't feel overly social.

That evening I realised it was probably time to get going. I had thought it would be nice to have the baby at a birthing centre instead of the hospital, so instead of a two-minute drive we had a 30-minute trip ahead of us, and I didn't want to leave it too long. The birthing centre provided lovely birthing rooms with birthing pools and no medical intervention. It also offered a private room where your husband could join you and your baby after the birth. I was of the opinion that hospitals were for when you were sick or broken, and childbirth didn't fit into either of these categories, unless something went wrong. Childbirth is a natural process, and I didn't want it to be over-medicalised. I decided against a home birth as we lived in flats at Bible College and there was very little privacy. The birthing centre seemed like the perfect compromise.

When the time came to leave for the centre, my husband decided he would be organised and put the rubbish bags out for the next morning, while I leaned impatiently and in deep pain against the car he had forgotten to unlock, wondering how he could be thinking of *rubbish bags* at a time like this. Once we were off, I looked at him and said, 'When we get back home again we'll have a baby!' I couldn't even imagine what that would be like.

We arrived at the birthing centre at around 7pm. Our baby girl was born at 10:28pm. Once labour got established, it went quickly and was straightforward. I had a water birth, and the pain was more than I had ever imagined was possible – it felt as though my body was being torn in two. Yet once my baby emerged from the water, I thought she was the most beautiful thing I had ever seen.

A rush of motherly love came like a tidal wave, washing away the darkness of depression in a moment of crashing and exultant freedom. It felt like midday. My joy was full; I could not have loved that baby more.

I lay in bed for what was left of the night staring at her, loving her. She weighed in at a petite 6.8lb and was perfectly formed. I knew my life had changed forever. I was a mother. It was amazing. We named her Piper Rose.

CHAPTER TWO

A Life Drained of Colour

The early days were fairly euphoric. She was a night screamer, so they were by no means easy. But I was so happy, and it was only now that I realised the depth of my ante-natal depression. Life now was beautiful. I watched my gorgeous daughter grow, and sorrow mingled with delight. I wanted another little baby; she was growing so fast. I would hold her over my shoulder, looking in the mirror in her room, and marvel at how much she had grown in such a short time. Those days of newborn joy and wonder and love I wanted again. The desire to have another baby overrode the dreadful memories of the pregnancy.

When Piper was only nine months old, I found out I was pregnant again. I was excited; I had wanted this – but then the memories of my last pregnancy came flooding back. I felt panicky; I almost wished I could undo it, make the pregnancy go away, but I couldn't. It felt surreal. I told anybody and everybody that I was pregnant, somehow thinking that if they knew it would make the pregnancy more real.

The nausea and vomiting came, and with it the despondency. It was not easy, having a baby to care for as well. I feel as though I missed out on enjoying my little girl for those nine months.

I had lost the ability to enjoy anything, even things I loved dearly. I didn't have the emotional capacity to feel joy, to take pleasure in the things I loved. I was there for all of it, but in a world drained of colour. To this day I don't even like looking at photos of her at that time; anything that reminds me of that period in my life brings an awful empty sort of pain.

I have to confess, I put up little resistance to my feelings. It would all go away the moment the baby was born, so I didn't try to fight the invasion of depression; I was just waiting until it was over. I carried on, my hope being in the birth, the end of suffering. I felt emotionally out of control, and I wondered how my husband could put up with being around me. I asked him once how he could stand it, and he said he loved being around me. I told him quite frankly that I didn't believe it, that I didn't even like being around myself (but I didn't have a choice). However, he never gave the impression he was fed up with me, nor was he anything other than a patient and loving husband.

At the end of the pregnancy I was again overdue. A full week went by and I was almost out of my mind. A friend made a joke about getting me a badge that read 'I love being pregnant'. She meant it lightheartedly, knowing I hated pregnancy. But it wasn't something I could laugh about. I wanted to drive off a cliff. I felt resentful towards this baby who simply wouldn't come. At my 41-week scan they told me the baby was going to be a full kilogram (two pounds) bigger than Piper. I went home and cried. It wouldn't come, and now it was enormous.

Labour finally came, not very consistently, but definitely there. My midwife was the same one I had had the first time – she was short, plump and easy-going, and told me I had lovely, easy births and that she would love to be my midwife again. She said the labour would most likely be half the time of my first, and when it came to the end it would just take a few pushes. By this calculation, I reckoned the labour should be over in three hours.

I went to the birthing centre again, I was in the same birthing room as last time, and I was hoping for the same kind of birth. Then it would be over. The darkness in my mind would be banished, leaving love and joy and delight in my new baby, just like last time.

I was a few hours in when I knew that things were definitely not the same as before. Longing simply to be free of pregnancy and in a desperate mental state, I couldn't understand why it was taking so long. I should have been pushing by now, and I thought I could feel the urge to do so, and yet I was nowhere near that stage. The midwife offered to break my waters to help speed things up. I agreed, not knowing that this would increase the pain. Being in a birthing unit, I had no pain relief available. They offered no intervention. The nearest hospital was a thirty-minute drive away.

I couldn't face being in the birthing pool. The pain was unbearable; I was dripping with sweat and I couldn't cope, yet there was no escape. I had been very resistant to the idea of a hospital birth, but now I wished I was there, so they could cut me open and end this pain. I was exhausted and at the end of myself, and still there was no escape.

The urge to push finally came. In a few pushes it would be over. And then – it was *not* over; I was having agonising contractions again. I knew this wasn't how it was supposed to be; I had done it before, and it wasn't like this. I pushed and pushed. He wasn't coming. The midwives were exchanging concerned looks. They decided to call the ambulance if he wasn't there by 12:40. My midwife performed an episiotomy (a local anaesthetic and small cut) to make it easier for the baby to come out. They called in an extra midwife.

My baby was born at 12:40. We named him Edward – Teddy for short.

CHAPTER THREE

Haunted by Trauma

I now had a baby boy, grey in colour, with long fingernails. *You just wouldn't come*, I thought, dispassionately, as they handed him to me. There was no rush of motherly love this time. Instead I felt numb and exhausted. I couldn't comprehend the birth experience I had just had, or the emotional damage it had caused me. I shut it in a vault so deep inside I did not even know it existed. In the absence of motherly love, I went through the motions of a mother who loved her baby. I knew what that was meant to look like.

I felt traumatised the next day. I asked my parents to wait a day before coming from out-of-town to see me. I couldn't face people. Bruwer had to take care of our daughter, and I was left sad and alone with a baby I didn't feel connected to at all.

Feeding didn't go well this time around, intensifying my sense of disconnect with my baby. Feeding was supposed to be a bonding time; I dreaded it. In the birthing centre they really pushed the notion of 'skin-on-skin' time for bonding. When they heard me say that I didn't feel attached to him they told me, 'You know what is great for that? Skin-on-skin time. Just put him on your chest and he will settle. He will keep warm. He can't get too hot or cold there. It really is the best thing.'

So I stripped off his tiny clothes, feeling flustered and stressed as he squirmed and cried. I put him on my chest, but he didn't settle. He continued to squirm and cry, and despite what the nurse said about temperature control, we both got hot and sweaty and began to stick to each other. It was awful. I stuffed his crying, wriggling body back into his clothes, and abandoned the so-called skin-on-skin time.

I *did* love him. In the following days at home I would look at him with a desperate, guilty sort of feeling. Although I had an instinctive motherly love and a desire to nurture and care for him, it was mingled with guilt – because I couldn't seem to find that passionate, fierce joy which would make that responsibility a delight.

I knew I had to fulfil the responsibility, and I was burdened for his welfare.

But small things started to go wrong. I caught conjunctivitis, and of course poor Teddy got it too. Getting eye drops into a newborn is not an easy job. It didn't take long for Teddy and I to learn this together. It was one more small stress when things were already strained. Then he developed very bad nappy rash. Then his breasts became swollen and infected. It is common for new babies to have swollen breasts due to the hormones, rarer that they become infected. In fact when I took him to the doctor and told him what had happened, his response was: 'I doubt it.' But upon taking a look he apologised and admitted I was right. A course of antibiotics followed. Yet another thing to force onto my baby. And all the while my guilty, desperate heart trying to find the love I heard him crying out for.

The first time I felt love towards him was during a feed, when I was giving him a bottle of expressed milk. He loved the bottle. I loved the bottle. I wished that I could give him a bottle all the time, but 'breast is best' had been drilled into me, and I felt too overwhelmed by guilt to do it. I longed for someone to tell me, 'Just put him on the bottle, it will be okay.' But no one did.

Then I began to have a recurring nightmare about him dying as a result of my leaving him in a hot car. I was irrationally fearful for him. I soon realised that I didn't like talking about the birth with people who came to visit and asked questions. I knew that with my first baby I had been happy to talk about the birth when asked. This time I didn't know what to do with how I felt, so I ignored my discomfort and answered their questions anyway. I answered as briefly as I could. What did it all mean? I just didn't know.

Those days were certainly not filled with the euphoric delight I had experienced with my first baby. They were hard. One night, after almost no sleep, a friend came over and offered to take Teddy for a while so I could sleep. I let her. I felt guilty, in that desperate way which had now become so familiar. She had him for about five hours and gave him a bottle feed. I had skipped a whole feed and had barely even noticed. He was only three weeks old.

Another time that same friend mentioned that she thought I had post-natal depression. I didn't agree. I knew that feeling of being depressed during pregnancy, like I was almost losing my mind, like I would do anything rather than be pregnant anymore. Now even the worst days were better than any day whilst pregnant. No, this didn't feel like depression. I felt numb. I felt traumatised.

Meanwhile my husband finished his theological studies, and we moved to a pastoral position at the other end of the country. The movers came and packed up our things, and the truck left. As we were doing the final cleaning of the house, Piper fell off the only piece of furniture left and needed stitches in her cheek. That was the beginning of a week of nightmarish proportions as Bruwer drove down to our new house and I stayed with my parents, later to fly down and meet him after he had arrived. I had a baby who wouldn't feed and cried from hunger. I had a toddler with a black eye, covered with insect bites, one of which got infected and swelled to the size of a tennis ball. Along with this she contracted a stomach bug and ended up in the emergency room in the middle of the night. It was a truly hellish time. At the end of it all I flew with my two babies down to the bottom of the country to start a new chapter of my life.

Nevertheless, it was a good life in many ways. We were living in a lovely old manse in a small rural town where it snowed in winter and everyone knew your name. My husband was doing what he loved, we had a lovely place to live in, and I had two wonderful children.

Two children. It never felt enough, like a complete family. We would have to have more.

The idea haunted me. I thought about it every day – not longingly, but with a tortured mind. Not a day went by that I did not think how glad I was not to be pregnant, and then came the thought that I would have to go there, coupled with the feeling that I couldn't bear facing it again.

Cracks began appearing. The first big crack I noticed one night at a ladies' dessert evening, when a woman was talking about the birth of her youngest child. It was the sort of birth story where everything went well, and I couldn't stand it. I felt as though I had to get away or scream. I excused myself with a light-hearted remark and went to the bathroom for a while. I looked at myself in the mirror and realised that these feelings weren't going away, and that they weren't normal. The months since Teddy's birth were passing by, but my feelings of trauma surrounding it were not. They were in fact getting worse.

One night whilst on the internet, I discovered the Trauma After Birth (TAB) website, and it was there that I finally found something that seemed to give a name and validity to what I was experiencing. It helped immensely to read about other women's stories and then to think through my own.

It was hard to go there. But one night I took the Holy Spirit's role as Counsellor literally, and decided to tell it to him from the beginning. I ran a hot bath, and I told him aloud the story of Teddy's birth, from the beginning. It was difficult to get through, and in parts I couldn't stop crying. But it was cathartic, and I felt better for some time after that. Something about putting into words all that had happened and telling it to Someone who was completely safe was a relief. In doing so the torment of the memory of it all lost some of its sting.

I continued to struggle with feelings of attachment to Teddy, however. He was mine, but he didn't really feel like mine. If someone had told me he had been swapped at birth I would have believed them, and it would have explained a lot. But I had been the only person in the birthing centre the night he was born, and he had never left my sight, so that explanation was not a possibility. It was hard having a baby who aroused no innate sense of joy and delight. I never looked at him with that unconscious feeling of enjoyment in the way I did with Piper. Had I not had that experience the first-time round, perhaps I would have found it easier to let the love take time to grow and the connection time to form. It was difficult knowing how amazing it had been when love and joy had arrived complete and in a moment, and then living with the kind of love that grows slowly through the wasteland of trauma and guilt. The first time

I sat down and played with him he was almost a year old. I had just never thought of or wanted to do it before. I built a tower of blocks; he knocked it down. It wasn't until we had played for a few minutes that I realised this had never happened before. It had taken nearly a year, but I was beginning to engage with and enjoy my son.

Teddy's first birthday was approaching, and I knew it was going to be hard. I didn't want to remember that birth at all, let alone celebrate the day. I found a path forward with this thought – I couldn't celebrate his birthday, but we could celebrate him. I worded the invitations carefully: 'Come and celebrate one year of Teddy with us.' I made him a cake in the shape of a candle, teddy bear biscuits and little sausages wrapped in pastry. We had party hats and sang 'Happy Birthday'.

The numbness I'd felt ever since he was born had become normal, as had the constant underlying guilt and desperation. But my anxiety about the anniversary of that day increased as the evening approached.

I dreaded that moment – exactly one year since he had been born. 'This time last year' haunted my thinking. When had it all been over? I knew it had been late at night, close to midnight. What was the exact time? I went to the other room and got out my maternity notes, my stomach tied in knots as I scanned through and found the time of his birth – 00:40. It was already over, almost twenty-four hours ago!

Relief flooded over me and the tension melted away as I stood in the big manse kitchen staring out the window and seeing the light spill out into the backyard. The moment which I had dreaded all day had passed unnoticed earlier that morning while I slept.

I knew this was a big one, this one-year anniversary. In the future, that horrific event would be obscured by the yearly celebrations we have covered it with. A party given for the life that had been created would make it harder to remember the things that had been broken.

It was some time shortly after his first birthday that I caught myself in that moment, the moment when I *knew* that my motherly love for Teddy was alive. I was looking out the window at my husband and the children playing together in the backyard. Piper was running around, and Teddy was on Bruwer's shoulders. I was looking at them, unconsciously enjoying their happiness. I found myself looking at Teddy and simply enjoying him. I had never before in moments like these looked at Teddy in delight. I had always looked at Piper, and until now only enjoyed and delighted in her. Now there I was looking at Teddy, simply because I loved him and delighted in him at that moment. It was a turning point for me. The latent motherly love finally had been born, and it slowly began to flow towards this little boy.

Although this healing flow began to fill the breach between my son and me, I still struggled with the idea of pregnancy. Not a day went by that I did not think about it, and it was an ongoing relief to wake up each day not pregnant.

Teddy was two when my love for him finally reached the full and fierce flood that I had waited so long to experience. It had been growing steadily all year, until on his second birthday I looked at him and knew suddenly and without a doubt that he was worth it. I could now look at him and experience the full joy in his being; the last shadows of doubt over his costly birth had disappeared in the sunshine of this motherly love which now filled my heart. He was worth it; I no longer held any feelings in my heart that the cost had been too high.

The fallout from the two years this love had taken to grow

meant I struggled sometimes to treat Teddy as the two-year-old he was, because my emotional connection with him was so new. I loved him like a newborn child. I didn't want him to move out of a cot and into a bed. I wasn't ready. In regard to his behaviour, I often responded to him as though he was still a baby rather than the intelligent two-year-old he had grown into. It wasn't intentional. I realised that I wasn't always being rational in my responses to him, and I struggled to find the right balance. As a baby he always had a particularly sad-sounding cry, and all I could think when I heard it was that he was crying because he hadn't been loved enough. Consequently, I couldn't bear the sound of his crying, and it has taken me a long time to respond with objectivity to his tears.

I also still have difficulty connecting his baby photos with the child he is today. The baby I nurtured and cared for has a vague and unreal quality about him compared to the child I now know and enjoy. He is an amazing, unique and beautiful person. I grieve that the trauma of pregnancy and birth meant I didn't get to enjoy this from the beginning. His baby photos are in an album, and although he was beautiful, I do not look at them very often.

Around the time leading up to Teddy's second birthday, my trauma about pregnancy once again became heightened. Just the thought of becoming pregnant again was enough to bring on nausea, headaches and extreme tiredness, all symptoms I usually experience in pregnancy – and all that while only *thinking* about it!

Yet it felt as if there was someone missing from our family. I have a distinct memory of looking at the beautiful laughing faces of my two children and thinking, 'There is someone missing.' It was such a strong feeling. We were missing a daughter, and her name was Scarlett.

We looked into adopting. I knew deep down though that all this was just avoiding the real issue. One morning at Bible Study my friends were discussing the upcoming birth of a mutual friend's baby. Sitting around the table in the room where we had our study, we were just having a bit of chat before we got started. This specific friend had had some medical complications which had led to her being recommended a caesarean section but, being her first baby, she wanted to try to give birth naturally. This talk was starting to make me feel tense and panicky, and I wanted to scream out, 'She should take the C-section!' I couldn't stand listening to it anymore. My heart was beating faster than normal; everything had a heightened sense of reality. I had to get out of there, and I went to another room for a while until the conversation was over and I had regained my composure.

I realised this could not continue. I could not always leave the room when people started talking about giving birth. I was at a stage of life where most of my friends were having babies. It was unavoidable. It had been almost two years since the trauma of my second birth experience, but my reactions to hearing about pregnancy and birth were getting worse, not better.

I decided that I needed to deal with this problem; that with the Lord and his Word I was going to face this thing called pregnancy and birth, and I was going to overcome it. I went to the store and bought a 'pregnancy journal'. I have it here beside me right now – brown cardboard cover; red spiral binding; coloured stars on the front and back.

I began my journal by writing out scriptures regarding childbirth and related topics. Throughout my next pregnancy, and after it, I continued to study and think over what the Bible really had to say about childbirth, and what that means for us individually today.

In addition to searching the Scriptures for foundational truths, I made an appointment with my doctor. I didn't know where else to start, and I thought at least she could point me in the right direction.

And so I found myself sitting in the green vinyl chair in her room, not sure where to begin. I began somewhere in the middle, emotion choking me when I came to Teddy's birth. She reached out her hand and told me to hold onto it. So, grasping her hand and through the tears, I talked about his birth, and life since then. She was kind and sensible, and referred me to a counselling service.

Contrary to expectation, however, I felt more sensitive towards pregnancy after this, rather than less so. I had to leave the room as soon as someone started talking about birth, instead of waiting and listening with my usual morbid fascination until anxiety overwhelmed me.

As my counselling appointment drew nearer I became increasingly tired, fearful and anxious. I felt as though I was about to open a dark cupboard and I was not exactly sure what I would find inside. I didn't want to seek the Lord, and yet at the same time I felt drawn to him.

The following verses became a rock I clung to in the darkness:

Fear not, for I have redeemed you, I have called you by name, you are mine.

Because you are precious in my eyes, and honoured, and I love you, I give men in exchange for you, peoples in exchange for your life. (Isaiah 43:1,4)

The Lord is my portion, says my soul, therefore I will hope in him. (Lamentations 3:24)

Once again I sat in the counsellor's office and told my story. Again I could not speak of Teddy's birth without crying. I shared my feelings of disgust and revulsion about pregnancy, at even the sight of a pregnant woman. The counsellor suggested asking God what he thought of pregnancy. 'I'm sure he doesn't think it is disgusting,' she said.

It seemed like sound advice. So I dutifully sat in bed one night, Bible and journal out. I hesitated. Then I looked at Bruwer, who was next to me, and burst out, 'I don't want to read my Bible! I don't want to ask God how he sees pregnancy because he will think it is wonderful, and then I'll be pregnant again!'

With that I burst into tears, and cried and talked incoherently for the next half hour about things I didn't even know I had been thinking. Finding pregnancy disgusting and abhorrent protected me from it, and the idea of suddenly thinking it was wonderful terrified me because if it *was* wonderful then I would *want* to be pregnant – and I could not face that. Without realising it, I was protecting myself from pregnancy by making it into something I shrank from in distaste. Without this feeling of abhorrence, I would be left vulnerable and afraid.

The next morning I opened my Bible to the only place I could really think of which spoke specifically about pregnancy – Psalm 139.

> I praise you, for I am fearfully and wonderfully made. Wonderful are your works; my soul knows it very well. (Psalm 139:14)

There it was. Not once, but twice. Wonderful. He *does* think it is wonderful. I laughed out loud when I read it. But I was still so very afraid of it.

It was around this time that I dreamed I had a baby. I gave birth to a girl. She was the most beautiful baby I had ever seen, with dark curly hair and big dark eyes. I was filled with love for her. It was a good dream.

Now I wanted another baby. That dark cupboard that had been filled with lies had now been flooded with truth, and I knew I wanted another baby with all my heart. I knew pregnancy would be hard, but I was willing to walk that path to have another child, and I was eager to start – perhaps because I feared that if I waited too long I would lose my nerve. I dug into God's Word, and kept putting my faltering trust in him. My feelings swung back and forth like a pendulum – now afraid of pregnancy and wanting to avoid it, then willing; wanting it despite being afraid. I was hanging on to Christ and his promises with a death grip, desperately hoping that my belief in his unfailing love would perhaps spare me the suffering that had been so much a part of pregnancy for me in the past.

Then one morning I did the test, and the line turned blue. I put it on the shelf and looked at it while I took a shower. I was pregnant and I was happy about it. I was also nervous and overwhelmed. I was going to have a daughter, Scarlett.

And I loved her.

CHAPTER FOUR

Hope of Redemption

I was determined to do battle for my mind this time, and not to give in to the negative thoughts and feelings which I had surrendered to the previous times. This time I would fight, and I would finish knowing I had done everything I could to believe the truth and to trust in Jesus – to finish strong.

Morning sickness with its nausea, vomiting and tiredness arrived as usual, but this time not as strongly as with the other pregnancies. If you were to read my journal, you would see that it was a time of intense ups and downs emotionally. But despite this there is a consistent theme of turning back to the scriptures and the Lord, and trusting him. There was depression, fear and discouragement, and then trust, peace and assurance. A lot of it was dependent on how much sleep and rest I had had the night before! There was also real joy in the life of my little unborn girl.

The nausea and tiredness were all but gone when my friend invited me on a prayer retreat, and I gladly accepted the invitation. A whole day without the children, simply focussing on the Lord, sounded like an amazing luxury. We met at a retreat centre on the edge of town, and sat together in a circle in a large room – relaxed, eyes closed and listening to the reading of Isaiah 53.

The words flowed over me soothingly, like water over pebbles. And then verse 12 leapt out at me, and spoke to me about my approaching delivery.

In the reflective time afterwards, I wrote the following in my star-covered journal:

> For you shall go out in joy and be led forth in peace; the mountains and the hills before you shall break forth into singing and all the trees of the field shall clap their hands. (Isaiah 55:12)

This scripture, for seemingly no reason, made me think of childbirth, this coming childbirth. While I cannot claim that God is going to give me a childbirth experience that is full of joy and peace and clapping of hands, I can take this: that this passage is about redemption, about God redeeming his people, a great and glorious day. But we have tastes of that great final redemption now, and I do believe that God can redeem my experience of birth. I believe that my child can be led forth in peace. Because I can have peace in him. This passage is an encouragement.

I realise that I felt betrayed by God in my last birth. I had prayed and begged God to let that baby come quickly, and daily he had said 'No'. And then, when it finally happened, it had been hideous.

I am afraid of that, of the daily, hourly, minute-by-minute wait for labour. Of asking God and not getting an answer. I want to know peace, for this baby to come into the world while I am at perfect rest in the Lord. I know this means letting go of control, of letting God bring it forth in his time. That is so hard. My mind says, 'What if?' What if it goes overdue? What if it gets too big? What if I don't cope in those dreaded fourteen days after my due date? Both my other babies have been overdue – what if God asks me to wait again? Will I still remain in perfect peace?

I guess if I really trust him, I will. If I am willing to let go of trying to control the situation, and know he is trustworthy and good and kind. I will be glad to be free of the burden. It is a heavy burden, but I am kind of attached to it so it is hard to give it to God.

Do not be anxious about anything, but in everything by prayer and supplication with thanksgiving let your requests be made known to God. (Philippians 4:6)

Those verses in Isaiah became a kind of banner over my pregnancy, a promise I clung to – God redeeming my birth experience of this daughter, this loved and wanted child. This birth would be different, and this was going to be a little girl I would love and adore. Peace, love, joy – my daughter Scarlett! I dreamed about those precious moments when I would gaze upon my newborn baby, overflowing with motherly love and wonder. Again from my journal:

I am struggling. I have a conflict of emotions rising inside me. I want to cry at one moment, the next tear and destroy. I am angry; I am repentant; I am despairing.

I get lost in this, and weighed down by the knowledge that I am responsible for my own actions, but at the same time I have this feeling that I am being taken over and controlled by emotions. I lash out at my husband, the person who treats me with unfailing kindness and love. I feel like a puppet trying to regain control of my strings but being flung this way and that.

It is as though all the sin in me rises up and grows into a monster. If I didn't know better, I would say it feels like I have a demon inside me. I hate it, but I can't get rid of it.

Then people ask, 'How are you?' and I want to laugh bitterly in their faces. I'm feeling terrible, but I can't tell them that.

Where is God in all of this? Lost somewhere in the bewildered, tearful rage that I flounder in. There are moments of clarity, and then days like this. This is becoming more common. And there are weeks and weeks stretching ahead of me like a burning wasteland.

I'm tired all the time. I struggle with the children, struggle to be patient and self-controlled, and struggle to keep up with the housework. The normal tiredness of pregnancy and having young children is magnified by the mental tiredness of this battle for my mind. It is probably that which tips me over the edge into not coping.

As I approached the halfway mark of my pregnancy, I began to feel increasingly anxious about the birth. We were now living in a different city, so I had different options – the choice of two birthing centres or the hospital. I lay in bed one night going through a mental tour of a birthing centre, trying to force myself to look at the options. We would meet in the reception area; other pregnant women would be there. They would greet us. They would talk to us about what to do on our arrival there. Next we would file into a birthing room. There would be a pool, a bathroom, a bed… I had to stop. I was almost in tears. I couldn't bear the thought of it.

Hope of Redemption

My Bible Study at that time happened to be centred on the issue of anxiety, and I felt convinced that my worry was wrong. God said, 'Do not be anxious about anything...' (Philippians 4:6) and there I was, anxious about that which I could not control. I had not been letting my fears drive me to God in faith; rather I had been lying there each night, letting them grow to outrageous proportions. Once again I acknowledged my need to God, impoverished of anything to offer, and find grace in my time of need. And that need was greater than I could have realised. God was about to take away what I *thought* I had, and give me instead what I never wanted.

The morning of my twenty-week scan arrived. A worship song had been replaying itself over and over in my head, so I now listened to it out aloud several times – it was victorious and triumphant, and the sound of it drowned my fears.

It wasn't the health of my baby that I worried about – I simply needed assurance that it was a girl. Of course, I *knew* it was. After all, my instincts had been right both times before. But I was still a little anxious as I drank a bad cup of coffee at the cafe before we went for the scan.

The radiographer did all the usual measurements and checks; it all looked normal. I didn't care; my only concern was that it was a girl. She didn't look for the gender of the baby until the end of the session, and at first it looked as though she wouldn't be able to see clearly enough. And then…

'It's a boy,' she said.

CHAPTER FIVE

The Emptying

My world instantly began crumbling around me, as though everything was breaking up and I was falling into nothingness. I managed to ask in desperation, 'Are you sure?'

'Yep. I could be wrong, but it's pretty obvious,' she replied.

Tears welled up and could not be stopped. I got out of there as soon as I could, and sat in the car waiting for Bruwer to follow with the DVD of the scan. The vault which had been sealed that day I gave birth to Teddy now split apart, and what came out overwhelmed me. I wept bitterly and could not stop. Later that day, tears still running down my face, I made the following entry in my journal:

> This was the child that I felt was missing from our family. As I looked at my children's beautiful faces at the dinner table, at play or in the car, I would feel as though one face was missing. I therefore overcame my fear of pregnancy, birth and the consequent lingering trauma, and here I was, pregnant again. I was carrying my missing child, the child I desperately wanted, the beautiful face that was missing from our family. Her name was Scarlett, and I loved her.

This time I hoped it would be different – the birth, those days of detachment afterwards. This time I was going to try to be better, to love this child even as it grew inside me. And to love it when it was born; to relive that same beautiful delight I had experienced in my newborn baby Piper. It would happen again this time because this was my precious, beautiful Scarlett, my baby who would redeem the whole pregnancy and birth experience; this baby whom I already so loved.

But she is not there. She never was. This baby is a boy.

At those three words, 'It's a boy' from the ultrasound technician, my world collapsed. I heard nothing else she said. Tears welled up and I couldn't stop them. My heart felt as if it had stopped beating, and I wish it had. I went out to the car and cried bitterly.

I have cried for most of the day. I can't seem to help the grief which wells up when I realise that this is really happening. We are having a boy.

I don't want a boy. I want a girl. It was always supposed to be a girl. She would complete our family. This is the last one; this was going to be the last pregnancy I was going to suffer through, and then this daughter would have been the crowning jewel. Now there is no daughter. And I don't want a son. There was never a son missing from the family. I don't want it to be again as it was with Teddy, and it is inconceivable to me that I could have a good birth experience with a boy. It is not a labour of love, for a start; and boys are big, you don't fall in love with them the moment they come out. I wanted it to be such a beautiful and precious time, and now it won't be. There will not be those moments of adoration and love between me and this baby.

They were for Scarlett, and now she is not there. I feel she has died, but it is worse – she never even existed.

I know I should have more faith in God and be able to surrender to his will, but I feel so much grief right now it is hard to see his plan. He knows all things; he knew how much I wanted a girl – and he said 'No'. I know he must have a reason; I know he is to be trusted. But I am grieving for the daughter that I wanted, that I loved, that I will never have; now I am to have a boy instead. I would almost rather not have any more children. In fact, if I had known before that it was definitely going to be a boy, then I would probably not have allowed myself to become pregnant again.

Does this sound awful? It is. What mother doesn't want their child because it is not the gender they wanted? It is terrible; but right now, it's true. I wish this was simply a nightmare – that I would wake up and find that I was not pregnant anymore and that I was not carrying a son that I do not want or love. It seems impossible that I could feel differently.

A particular verse came to mind that day:

> 'For my thoughts are not your thoughts, neither are your ways my ways,' declares the Lord. 'For as the heavens are higher than the earth, so are my ways higher than your ways and my thoughts than your thoughts.' (Isaiah 55:8,9)

This verse was from the same chapter in Isaiah as the verses about redemption, which had become the banner over my approaching birth. It comforted me to an extent. I knew God was in this, that he had plans, and this helped as I wrestled through it.

The fear of giving birth escalated after I found out I was to have a boy. My midwife, concerned at the fact I was constantly in tears at appointments, referred me to the Maternal Mental Health Service. They came regularly to visit throughout my pregnancy, and the student who was working with my case worker was a Christian who offered free counselling sessions as part of her work experience. She would often come and sit at the kitchen table with me, the children parked in the other room in front of the TV, and we would talk about my fears and my anxiety around the approaching appointments. We discussed ways to make life easier, such as making use of online grocery shopping, and not worrying so much about the housework. It was helpful to simply talk about things with someone who understood what I was struggling with. It made me feel it was normal, that I wasn't the only one who had these struggles. These suggestions made me feel as though I had some kind of safety net around me – in case I fell off the cliff.

We talked long about this being a boy, and about what that meant for the birth. I knew even as I was saying it, that it was irrational to presuppose that because this was a boy, the delivery would not be a good experience. But something in my mind would not separate having a boy from the likelihood of a hard birth and not being able to bond. The lack of bonding was something I struggled much with – I wanted so much to love this baby, to cherish those sweet and precious moments with it as a newborn. The thought of having of that taken away from me and having it replaced with two years of struggling to bond was gut-wrenching and unbearable. I couldn't face it, so I tried to shut off my feelings of horror about the impending birth and what would likely follow, though it continued to hold me in its frightening grip. The trauma of my last pregnancy and this one were welded together in my mind; it didn't matter how irrational I knew I was being, I was unable to separate them emotionally; it was as though the reasoning process inside me had been broken. I could not conceive of being able to love a newborn boy, nor of enjoying his babyhood.

One day my counsellor asked me what I considered a 'successful birth experience' would look like, stressing how important it was for me to have this in mind. I answered that it would be a natural birth, one that I would handle well (meaning I would not feel out of control emotionally or physically), that labour would progress well, and that it would be quick. I was, without realising it, describing Piper's birth.

She looked at me thoughtfully and said, 'Could it not simply be that you *birthed*?'

It had never occurred to me that it could be as simple as that. That simply *giving birth*, in whatever form that came, could be a good and successful birth. It felt as if someone had just lowered the goal post to a point where I was guaranteed to get the ball over.

Yet despite victory in this arena, there were other battles still raging. For example, I struggled to know how to talk about the pregnancy with others, as the following excerpt from my journal indicates.

> It is hard to talk about this pregnancy. Since finding out we are having a boy, I have felt less and less comfortable talking about it. I'm scared they will ask what we are having. I dread the question because either way it exposes the fragility of my emotions. If I do not tell them then they will think I am keeping a delightful secret to share joyfully when the child is born. If I tell them, they will be glad for

me, which I could not stand; it would be so out-of-place with my unbearable feelings of grief. I told someone today, and tried to explain some of the reasons why this was not a joy and excitement to me. But the words were inadequate. How can you put into words what you do not understand yourself?

How do you describe this overwhelming grief, mingled with the comforting presence of God's goodness and love? I am not rejoicing over this unborn son, yet I do not hate him. I have a clear sense that he is cherished and loved, yet those feelings do not come from me. I cannot think of him without wanting to cry; I cannot imagine holding him in my arms and being overwhelmed by love for him. Yet I cannot truly say he is not wanted. I feel too strongly the power of God's plan, his inevitable force of love bringing this child into the world. He was not wanted by me, but he is wanted, planned, created and loved by God. Perhaps I am almost a little in awe of this baby. He represents something I don't understand – God's sovereign plan.

But all of these things are wound together with a grief and sorrow over the loss of our daughter Scarlett. She becomes less and less real to me, which does not lessen the grief, but only makes it more secret and isolating.

In all this I really wanted to understand the root of my birth trauma, and the intense fear and anxiety around it. I realised that there was a deep unwillingness in me to go through a bad birth experience again. I was not willing to accept that from the hand of the Lord. But at the same time I had no ultimate control over what would happen. I could, like the last time, do everything possible to be ready for the birth, to help it come, to labour well, but it *could* still go horribly wrong. It had done so last time – God's hand had dealt me a labour that I still suffer the effects of today. I was terrified about what he would do this time.

How do you reconcile that the One you are taking comfort and refuge in is the same One who allowed you to go through terrible pain and suffering, and that he might allow it again? It might be his hand who saves and upholds, but it is also his hand which crushes and afflicts.

Trusting him scared the heck out of me. But he was my portion and, like the apostle Peter, to whom else would I go? So, I put my hope in him.

Psalm 55 expressed my heart so well:

Give ear to my prayer, O God, and hide not yourself from my plea for mercy!
 Attend to me, and answer me; I am restless in my complaint and I moan...
 My heart is in anguish within me; the terrors of death have fallen upon me.
 Fear and trembling come upon me, and horror overwhelms me...
 But I call to God, and the Lord will save me.
 Evening and morning and at noon I utter my complaint and moan, and he hears my voice.
 He redeems my soul in safety from the battle that I wage... Cast your burden on the Lord, and He will sustain you; He will never permit the righteous to be moved (Psalm 55:1-2; 4-5; 16-18;22)

I came up with an analogy for pregnancy. People say it's 'only' nine months, and I appreciate that it seems to pass quickly when you are not the one who is pregnant. But pregnancy is like having to walk nine kilometres to your destination while everyone else is taking the bus. It is not far at all when you are the one on the bus, but it is very far when you are the one pregnant and walking alone. And what is most infuriating is when people on the bus think they can offer advice or encouragement. 'Not far to go!' 'You are looking great!' 'Such a precious time!' 'It'll be over soon.'

23 May 2011. I have a friend who lost her baby recently. She was 15 weeks pregnant. I felt awful. Here she was grieving for her child that she wanted and loved, and here I was carrying a living baby that I have not wanted because it is not a girl. I feel very small and childish. Right then I made a decision to love him, not despite the fact he is a boy but because of it. It is easier said than done.

3 June 2011. Something happened today. Something so small and yet so completely amazing. It was something from God, an answer to prayer. A miracle, a moment where everything changes in an instant.

We were leaving the pharmacy, the one right next door to the radiology clinic where I heard those words, 'It's a boy', and my heart turned to stone towards this baby. I had come through the tears, the questioning and the grieving, to acceptance – but not to joy or excitement or anticipation. As we drove out of the car park towards the exit, past the clinic, I saw a lady holding a little baby over her shoulder. He wore a baby-blue hat and a blue-and-white onesie. And something inside me grew warm and I thought how cute he was. Then I thought of our baby boy and imagined him being tiny and cute and my loving him.

I imagined loving him!

I thought of his presence in this world, and in our family, with pleasure and warmth and excitement. For the first time I truly felt as though I could enjoy and love him. It was amazing.

That was the moment when the experiences from my previous pregnancy and birth became separate in my mind from this present one.

I struggled in those last weeks – I was weary of the battle; I became self-absorbed because it took everything I had to get myself through the basic tasks of the day. Even cooking the dinner overwhelmed me; trying to get my thoughts in order simply to go through the steps of making a meal was too much for me. I would stand there just feeling completely overwhelmed by it. We ate a lot of toast for dinner at that time.

I was not a good mother in those days. In fact, I have trouble recalling the children much at that time, and I feel as though I lost a year of their lives. I was just in survival mode and there they were at two and four, growing up, and I couldn't enjoy them.

Looking back through my writing at the time, it is incredible to me that in those last difficult weeks and days I managed to record in my journal not only the writhing of a tortured mind, but also evidence of a peace and joy which could honestly praise the Lord.

I reached my due date in a state of peace, excited to meet the baby. My midwife had said she would refer me for induction at forty weeks instead of forty-one (which is usual practice), as part of the plan to make things manageable at the end. I really hung out for that. But of course, after the referral you often have to wait up to a week get an appointment. I was due on a Tuesday, but by now my appointment at the hospital to 'talk about booking an induction' was not until the *following* Monday morning.

At two days overdue I was struggling with the feeling I had been betrayed by God once again. I had prayed and prayed to be spared that agonising wait, and here I was once more not knowing when it was going to end. Once again those days stretched ahead of me – of waiting and waiting, with nothing happening. It made it harder that I had a lot of Braxton Hicks contractions in the two weeks leading up to my due date, some so strong they woke me up in the night; and yet there was no labour, no baby. I didn't understand why God would not let the baby come. I complained; I was bitter.

I read from the Psalms:

> When my soul was embittered, when I was pricked in heart, I was brutish and ignorant; I was like a beast toward you. Nevertheless, I am continually with you; you hold my right hand. (Psalm 73:21-23)

I am so glad the Bible has verses like that, ones which express your heart so perfectly, and comfort you by reminding you of the Lord's faithfulness. The next day, Friday, I started by comforting myself with the reading of the rest of Psalm 73, and praying that the baby would come, struggling to understand the wisdom of God's timing. According to my journal, that is how the day started; it finished very differently.

I received a phone call later that morning from a close friend whose baby had been due at the same time as mine. She had already delivered her baby, and I was truly glad for her. I hoped all day that I too would have my baby that day. But evening came and there was no sign of its arrival. I texted her with my congratulations and enquired as to how she was doing. Her reply ended with 'we are a very happy family', and immediately something inside me snapped. They had a baby; they were very happy. I sat here pregnant, with no baby, and not happy. It felt as if it was never going to happen.

I began a slippery descent into despair. I had not kept strong in my faith; I hadn't finished in perfect peace. I wasn't supposed to be like this; I was supposed to have done better this time around. I had tried so hard and failed. Why hadn't God intervened? I had prayed and begged him to give me this baby before it reached this point, and he hadn't. I felt frantic, as though I wanted to rip my stomach open and pull the baby out myself. I wished we had not decided to have another baby. I had no peace and no joy. It was supposed to be different this time.

The next day dawned, and I looked at it with eyes that did not see or care. It was Saturday, but I didn't get out of bed. I sat there; the children and my husband were moving around me, but they felt distant and removed. I just didn't care. I didn't care about any of it. I couldn't bring myself to get up, to stop crying, and to carry on with another day of being pregnant. I had an overwhelming sense of failure. I had wanted to be strong to the end, and had failed. I couldn't do it. I had tried to cling to God, to focus on his Word and to cling to the truth, but I had failed spectacularly.

I tried to think of a way to cope with what was happening, and whilst in the shower I hit on what I thought was just the thing.

'Hey, Bruwer,' I called to my husband, 'let's leave the kids with Mum and Dad for the weekend and go out of town and stay somewhere really nice.'

He smiled at me as though the idea appealed and he was indulging me, but then he said, 'But we can't – you might have the baby.'

The light died in my eyes and I replied in something between a hiss and a shout, 'But I'm *not* having the baby, am I? That's the point!'

I couldn't explain it – I knew it was crazy – but I couldn't just go on pretending that I was going to have a baby any minute. The constant expectation of release from this body of suffering, together with the constant disappointment that the baby would not come, was unbearable.

Bruwer, ever kind and patient, was getting to the end of *his* patience. When I suggested that he take the children out because I didn't want them to be around me in that state, he suggested somewhat shortly that maybe *I* should go out, since *I* was the one with the problem. Although this seemed reasonable, I knew I couldn't do it. I knew that if I got into a car, the most appealing thing in the world would be to find a quiet spot by the river and just drive in. To sink into oblivion in the murky waters of Lake Karapiro was frighteningly attractive.

This scared me. What was happening to me? Desperate, I called the number for the crisis line that Maternal Mental Health had given me. As I cried as I talked, and the young man with a British accent on the other end of the line did his best to help – with all the generic things they say to people who say they are feeling desperate and suicidal. He asked when I'd had the baby, and I explained that I hadn't, and that was the problem. He suggested some relaxation techniques, such as trying to ground myself, and making space to be alone but at the same time being around people. It all meant nothing to me, but part of me remotely appreciated the humour of the situation. He seemed to be at a loss with what to do with this emotional, sobbing, pregnant woman.

'What medication are you on?' he asked.

'I'm not on anything,' I quavered, trying to sound less hysterical. 'I'm really very normal when I am not pregnant.' That must have been hard for him to imagine!

I stood in the baby's room – there was the baby hammock, clean and made up for him; the day bed with its pile of cushions; the white drawers filled with baby clothes, carefully washed and folded; the changing table, ready with nappies and wipes. There was everything I needed, except the baby. I was filled with rage at this unfulfilled expectation, my fists clenched, longing to tear that bed apart, to overturn the change table, to throw it all in the wardrobe and scream. We were expecting a baby and he hadn't come. I didn't want him to come with me in a state like this. I wanted to be able to look forward to his arrival when I had at least some semblance of peace and joy in Christ. This was supposed to be the redeeming birth, the one where I didn't give in to this sort of despair, the one where I could say I had fought the fight and finished the race. *I had failed.*

CHAPTER SIX

The Bottom of the Pit (Where Jesus is Found)

Out of the chaos the phone rang, and I answered it automatically. I love talking on the phone, even in the state I was in, and the temptation to find out who wanted to speak to me was irresistible. It was a friend who had known me since we were five, who went through school with me, and who had suffered through pregnancies too. She normally lived with her family overseas, where they served as missionaries, but now just 'happened' to be home on furlough. She was calling to ask if we would like to meet her family at the lake. Although I was not able to even talk to her without crying, it seemed like something I could manage. I don't think I could have borne anyone else, but I *could* face an outing with her.

Through this interaction I had made contact with the world around me, and I began to function once again with a semblance of normality. I stopped crying. I got the family ready to go out, and we stopped to get something to eat on the way. It took supreme effort on my part to do any of this as it felt like I had already failed, that nothing I could do would change the fact that I had not endured until the end. I had not stayed strong in my faith; my spirit was broken.

The trip to the lake was good. I remember not having much to say to my friend, but she didn't seem to mind; I don't know if anyone else would have been quite as easy to be with at this time. In the midst of my distress, God was showing his grace to me through this ordinary outing.

We went home with plans to have dinner with them that night. It kept me sane, having to socialise, having to be with other people.

There was still Sunday to live through, before Monday and the opportunity to go to the hospital in the hope of action. I did not expect to go into labour before then. I felt an unreal sense of calm – not exactly peace, more a sense of surrender. I was like someone who had fought to keep from slipping to the bottom of a pit, but, having failed to do so, had no reason to keep fighting.

Monday morning came, and with it the appointment to 'talk about induction'. I wanted to pray that the staff would be favourable towards me, that they would understand how important it was to get the baby out. But I didn't know what to ask for, so I prayed something like this:

'Jesus, I don't even know how to pray, because I have prayed for so many things lately that I thought were good things, and you said 'No'. But I am in the habit of asking you for help, so here I am.'

The hospital and maternity ward no longer held terrors for me – my only terror was a continued pregnancy. I sat in a shared room full of equipment and was hooked up to a machine to be monitored. The nurse started to talk about the possibility of being induced, and I began to cry.

'You don't want to be induced?' she asked.

'No, I really do,' I answered, my voice small and tight with tears. 'I just feel like I would rather do anything than be pregnant anymore, like getting into the car and driving into the river is a really good idea.'

She passed me some tissues, drew the curtain around me, and disappeared for a while. I sat there, huge, snivelling and humiliated that I had sounded suicidal. It wasn't entirely true; I didn't *want* to die, it was just that I couldn't face being pregnant anymore, and so the oblivion of sinking into the murky depths of the river was appealing in comparison. If sounding suicidal was what it took to make them understand that I needed to be induced, I was willing to let them know. At the bottom of the pit, you have nothing left to lose.

I was led into a private room for an ultrasound. The doctor came in. I had imagined myself pleading my case to an unsympathetic middle-aged man, but instead I found myself in the hands of a sweet and sympathetic young woman.

'I hear you've been having a hard time,' she said to me.

I found myself telling her about how I felt like tearing my stomach open with a knife, just to get the baby out. I dampened several more tissues. She finished the ultrasound and said, 'I think we should induce you today, and I think you should have an early epidural to help you stay calm.'

A weight was lifted off my shoulders. From that moment, the desperate despair was gone. I was going to have the baby *today*.

My maternal mental health worker came to see me while I waited in the tiniest room imaginable before going upstairs for the induction. I had some magazines for company, accompanied by sounds of severe distress and pain from an unseen patient down the corridor. Although I was feeling better, I was glad when she arrived. I still felt ashamed that I had got to breaking point, that I hadn't coped. She was the only person who treated me as though I were normal. She understood that merely entertaining the thought of driving into the river was an appealing idea, distinctly different from actually intending to do it.

'Everyone has thoughts,' she said, 'but there is a difference between thoughts and intentions'.

When I told her about wishing we were not even having a baby anymore she said, 'But if I gave you a magic wand, and you could just wave it and all of this would go away and you wouldn't have a baby, would you do it?'

Slowly I shook my head. 'I wouldn't.'

So, I guess, I really did want that baby.

Smiling and encouraging, she said to me, 'I wouldn't say this if it wasn't true – I honestly think that you have handled this brilliantly.'

I looked at her in frank disbelief. In what universe could this ever be called handling something brilliantly?

'I'm serious,' she said, reading my face. 'Look, you called the crisis line and you gave them my number when you got here. Now you are here, about to have the baby. You did all the right things.'

I couldn't see it then: the sense of failure was too great. All I saw was the failure and shame of not coping. I still held on to that ideal, that I had intended to 'do better' this time. My feeling of not having coped implied failure – which, after the long battle, was a bitter defeat.

I spent the next few hours in an old, run-down ward, hoping the gel they applied to my cervix would get the contractions started. During this time Bruwer and I walked around, got ourselves a variety of overpriced foods from the cafeteria, and climbed up and down a dimly-lit stairwell. I was having some contractions – but I had been having them off and on for weeks, and I was reluctant to rest in case they stopped altogether. While

Bruwer went home to get the laptop so we could watch a movie, I opened up my Bible, not knowing what to read. The light was so dim it was difficult to read the words, and I didn't know which of the multiple switches on the wall was the light; I was wary of accidentally setting off some kind of alarm. So I read the first thing I saw on the page. It was the account of Jesus praying in the Garden of Gethsemane before his crucifixion.

As I read it became clear to me, as never before, that here Jesus was praying for something he knew could never happen. Just as I had prayed earnestly for this baby to be born naturally and on time, and that I would be spared this anguished despair of hope disappointed, so Jesus had prayed to be spared from the agony of a wrath he did not deserve. And as he prayed, he knew the answer would be 'No'. He prayed that not his will but rather the Father's will be done. He, more than any other person ever, knew the anguish of a prayer unanswered, of a request denied. He was my example, as in the face of bearing the horrors of the sins of all mankind he prayed, 'Not my will, but yours be done.'

Despite my sin and failure, so very different from the perfect life of my Saviour, I felt a sense of fellowship with Jesus; he too had walked this path of suffering that I now walked. 'I know,' he told me, 'I know. I prayed too, and the answer was no. I suffered too.'

I sat in that horrible little hospital room, not yet in labour, and honestly and sincerely praised Jesus for what he had done and was doing for me; knowing that he would be with me, holding my right hand, loving me and redeeming me.

By 8pm I was in labour. The midwife came in and took me down to the delivery suite, which was in a lower floor of the building. Progress was interrupted as I regularly stopped to grip the handrail during contractions, unable to move. Shortly after we got to the delivery suite, she broke my waters. As had been the case with Teddy, the contractions soon became unbearable. Knowing that I was not anywhere close to giving birth, I asked for an epidural. I could not believe that I had given birth twice before with pain like this. It was horrendous, and with each contraction I just kept thinking about the epidural, and that it would be over soon; it felt like such a long time before it was set up and actually working. It felt surreal when I eventually was sitting on the hospital bed in a hospital gown, wires and tubes coming out of me, hooked up to machines. How different from the other births! I knew I was doing the right thing to ensure this baby would arrive that day, using all the help I could get. It felt incredible as the pain wore off completely. I knew my body was going through agony, but I was feeling none of it, and I wondered why more people didn't choose to have epidurals.

I dozed a little. I could feel the baby moving down, and when they examined me, they said they could see his head and it was time to push. It took longer than I had expected, to push that little baby such a short distance. They had called in the doctor to use some tool to help get him out, but I thought, 'No way are you sucking my baby out!' and I used everything I had to push him out before the doctor got there.

And then he was there. I had a brief moment of thinking how alien-like it was to have a living thing being pulled out of my body. And then I had him on my chest. Little, alive and mine. How I loved him.

He must have stayed on me for a couple of hours while the epidural wore off. He fell asleep on my chest and I looked at him, thinking how adorable he was. It was all over; my baby was mine, and I was his.

My midwife came in just before I was ready to leave the delivery room. She told me she thought I should stay at the hospital, that there was a room prepared for me. She assured me that I wouldn't have to share, but would have my own room. She insisted that she really thought it was best that I stayed, that she wasn't happy for me to leave so soon.

My state of calm was giving way to a rising feeling of stress. The thought of having to stay in hospital was appalling; Bruwer would have to leave and I would be left all alone in a dingy hospital room. There was no way that I was going to do that.

'But I don't want to stay here,' I cried, 'I am going to the birthing centre!'

'I think it would be better for you to stay here, even just for the day. If you think about it, it was just a couple of days ago that you were feeling… you know. What are you going to do if you are at the birthing centre and if you start to feel like that again?'

I stared at her, realising that she really had not understood. 'But I am fine now,' I insisted, 'I'm not pregnant anymore, I'm fine.'

And it really was *that* simple. I was not pregnant anymore. I was sleep-deprived and exhausted, but I was me again. I knew I was no danger to myself or my baby. The problem had been being pregnant – now that was over and I was fine.

I won. She let me go. I spent the day at a birthing centre vainly trying to rest. After dinner we came home and it was lovely – just Bruwer, Billy and I for the next three days. I curled up on my own couch to watch TV and slept in my own bed, finally getting some rest, my husband and baby both with me.

It turns out you *can* love baby boys. You can look at their tiny perfection and simply adore them. God gave me another son, and I love him.

Those early days were a time of adjustment in many ways. For several days I struggled to shake off those lingering feelings of disappointment in my failure, until I slowly began to realise how much more evident God's grace was in my weakness.

I felt like a spring that had been coiled as tightly as possible for a long time, and then suddenly released. For a while I seemed to bounce around, reeling in the freedom from strain, before settling down into a normal rhythm. I felt the freedom of no longer being centred on myself, because it had taken all my mental and emotional resources up to now to cope with each moment of each day. After being released from this necessity, it took me some time to readjust. Life was hard and overwhelming, but in a normal way. It was hard because I had three preschoolers and one of them was a newborn. It was hard because I had these little ones with me all day, every day. It was hard because I was physically exhausted and felt the demands on me required too much sacrifice. But all this was simply motherhood, and despite the struggles I was able to function like myself again. Many days I wanted to put my head down and cry, but every single moment of every day was better than those whilst being pregnant. This was what I wrote in my diary at that time:

> 27 November. I didn't know it could be like this. I didn't know a baby boy could bring so much joy. I could never have known or believed it unless God had shown me. He knew. As he removed my dream of a much-loved and wanted daughter, as he walked with me through the grief and loss, the fear and pain, he knew. He knew that the only way to heal the wound I carried was to give me another son. He knew that a redemptive birth was one that did not avoid the horror of the last one, but rather one in which I was forced to face it with a growing joy and peace I never

believed possible. I am grateful that he loved me enough not to give me what I wanted. I am grateful that he loved me enough to walk with me through the pain so that I could discover that all I need is him.

PART TWO

Babies and the Bible

In Part One I shared my experiences of pregnancy and childbirth. Throughout my third pregnancy I studied what the Bible had to say on the subject. I discovered that there is a surprising lack of Christian material (none, in fact!) to help women going through difficulties in their pregnancies. I hadn't been helped by the usual 'birth is God's wonderful design' attitude. What I experienced *wasn't* wonderful – it was extreme suffering.

We read in Genesis:

> To the woman he said, 'I will surely multiply your pain in childbearing; in pain you shall bring forth children. Your desire shall be for your husband, and he shall rule over you.' (Genesis 3:16 NASB)

Although there is much written about the second half of that verse, no one seems to say much about the 'childbearing' part. It is as though we all assume the meaning is obvious – giving birth hurts. Although God's design is wonderful, childbirth is specifically identified as being part of the curse. What does this mean?

Childbearing Redeemed

Does the Word have any relevance to my suffering at all? And to the suffering of others? I came to the conclusion that it does, and the following part of this book is the result of my studies. I hope that you will be encouraged by the themes of childbirth and redemption which I trace through the Bible and which find ultimate meaning in the cross.

CHAPTER SEVEN

The Blessing and the Curse

I have climbed mountain peaks that gave me views of glaciated mountains in wave after waves of ranges, but none of those breathtaking vistas was comparable to seeing that baby enter the world; I have heard the most delicate and exquisite birdsong and some of the best musicians in the world, but no sounds rivalled the cries of that baby.

– Eugene Peterson [2]

What God created was good.

I suppose I had always held on to the vague idea that the story of childbearing began in Genesis 3:16, which (as we have seen) says:

> To the woman he said, 'I will greatly multiply your pain in childbirth, in pain you will bring forth children; yet your desire will be for your husband, and he will rule over you.' (NASB)

But to understand more fully God's design and purpose, and

allow ourselves to be mentored through childbearing by his Word, we must go further back, to where the Bible starts with the wonderful account of God creating the world and everything in it. His final creation was of man and woman in his own image. They were given the ability to 'multiply', and out of their perfect, shameless union was the potential for an ever-growing community of people made in the image of God. He designed a woman's body to conceive, carry, give birth to and nurture another small human being. This is a beautiful and amazing design, one by which life gives birth to life and so continues God's creation.

The gift of children was a blessing bestowed on Adam and Eve by God:

> And God blessed them. And God said to them, 'Be fruitful and multiply and fill the earth and subdue it, and have dominion over the fish of the sea and over the birds of the heavens and over every living thing that moves on the earth.' (Genesis 1:28)

This was God's purpose for us: to bear children and fill the earth with people created in God's image, who would work in the world God had created, subdue it and have dominion over it. This purpose, as in all of God's creation, was good. In fact, God says it was 'very good!'

But creation did not stay very good. Eve was deceived by Satan, and Adam followed her into sin. They became spiritually dead. The perfect relationship they had enjoyed with God was ruined, and their sin led to condemnation for all humanity yet to be born. Creation had become subject to futility and decay.

But God did not take away the blessing of bearing children.

In fact, God said that it was through the bearing of children that one day the Saviour would come and redeem humanity and the world, and that he would 'bruise the serpent's head' (Genesis 3:15). The advent of this future Saviour would ultimately result in the crushing blow to the ancient serpent, who is called the devil and Satan, freeing creation from the curse it had become subject to.

While childbirth was always part of God's blessing, it now also becomes a symbol of hope and of a future Saviour. Yet the third chapter of Genesis is filled with sorrow and loss:

> …therefore the LORD God sent him out from the garden of Eden to work the ground from which he was taken. He drove out the man, and at the east of the garden of Eden he placed the cherubim and a flaming sword that turned every way to guard the way to the tree of life. (Genesis 3:23-24)

Cursed, ashamed and cut off from the Lord, Adam and Eve are driven from their home, unable to return. As we look around our world, appalled at the evil and suffering we see, consider what it must have been like for Adam and Eve after they had known a world where suffering and evil did not exist? How could they bear to live cut off from God, with whom they had lived in an untainted relationship? How could they still have hope in life?

The next verse tells the story of hope, of God's grace in their life, the evidence that he is still blessing them even in this broken creation.

> Now Adam knew Eve his wife, and she conceived and bore Cain, saying, 'I have gotten a man with the help of the LORD.' (Genesis 4:1)

Eve recognised God's hand in the conception and birth of her son, and she knew this blessing was from the Lord.

Children are seen as a blessing throughout the Bible narrative. The shame and stigma of not bearing children was deep and painful, as is seen in the examples of Rachel and Hannah. To have children, and especially to have many children, was to be blessed. In a world of sickness, violence and death, life was precarious. The more children you had, the less chance there was of getting to old age and having no one around to care for you. In a world without the pension, retirement, or Aged Concern, children were your old-age plan and security. There are cultures where this is still the norm.

> Children are a blessing and a gift from the LORD. Having many children to take care of you in your old age is like being a warrior with a lot of arrows – the more you have, the better off you will be, because they will protect you when your enemies attack with arguments. (Psalm 127:3-5 CEV)

When we look at Scripture, there is no doubt that children are to be recognised as a blessing. In the Old Testament they could be seen as a sign of hope, of looking forward to the One who would crush the enemy. God would keep his promise – the woman would bear children; her seed would ultimately defeat Satan. God had not forsaken his people.

After the birth, death and resurrection of Christ, we are still given the blessing of children. We have the opportunity to introduce our children to Jesus and all he has done for them. We see in children not only the hope that God will keep his promise, but joy that he has done so.

CHAPTER EIGHT

In Pain

Wanting the blessing of a child is one thing. The reality of the pain which results from bringing a child into the world is another thing altogether. Pregnant with my first child, I remember older women with children of their own trying to make me aware of the pain of childbirth. I heard them, but I couldn't really know how bad it could be. I thought such things as: 'Well, it doesn't kill you, or go on forever! How bad can it really be?' Of course, the reality is that childbearing can result in death, and even when it doesn't, it brings pain which words are inadequate to describe.

It seems to me that when it comes to the way we Christians deal with the pain of childbearing, two main approaches compete for our attention in this modern world.

The *first* view is that the many forms of pain relief and intervention which enable us to give birth with less pain and fewer mortalities are evidence of God's common grace. These modern medical advances are to be accepted as a gracious gift from the Lord, and they diminish the effects of the curse. Childbirth does not need to be so painful anymore. The *second* view downplays the curse and the fallen condition of our current age. This view calls us to allow birth to be as natural as possible – because 'pain has a purpose', and is therefore not something to be removed but instead worked with and embraced. Your body has natural ways of dealing with pain and these are ideally not to be interfered with. It is expected that childbirth will be uncomplicated in most cases where nature is allowed to follow its course.

I would suggest that both of these views attempt to minimise the reality of pain in childbirth, but in different ways. One is to alleviate the pain with modern medicine; the other is to accept the pain by believing nature to be essentially good. Both can be helpful – and harmful.

Natural childbirth is rising in popularity among Christian women. They believe that one should let go of the fear and embrace the presence of God in one's experience. They suggest one should invite Jesus into the whole experience, and with his presence navigate the rough waters of childbirth without anguish, suffering, sorrow or fear, but rather with his peace and joy. They maintain that our bodies were made to do this, so we can approach childbirth with confidence in God's design and purpose.

It is a good and godly thing to embrace the truth that Jesus is intimately with you in childbirth, and in the months of pregnancy. To seek him and rely on him for strength and grace each day, especially in the hardest of times, is indeed a great comfort. But it will not exempt you from suffering. Women do not suffer in childbearing simply because they are afraid or are not trusting the Lord sufficiently. Removing fear may help the birth process, but it will not ensure a pain-free or easy one. Women suffer in childbirth because we are giving birth in a broken world, and this process is not immune from it. A Christian view of childbirth must exist in this reality, where brokenness and suffering are the norm. Straightforward births are a gift of grace and mercy. The fact that childbearing so often goes well is a gracious, but imperfect, reminder of God's original design.

In countries where women give birth without access to medical care, the death rate is high. I recently spoke with a nurse who worked in a mission hospital in South Sudan, and who has witnessed the everyday reality of women and babies dying in childbirth. Without access to medical care, women in such circumstances give birth naturally, without intervention, and many of them die. There, people have no illusions about childbirth being a beautiful, peaceful and joyful thing. Rather, it is dangerous and death is normal. She told me the tragic account of a mother who watched her daughter die in childbirth and who was not surprised by the outcome. Rather, she was surprised that the hospital staff even tried to save her daughter's life! Like in so many places, death was the expected and unsurprising outcome of childbirth.

However, some people struggle to accept that childbearing is deeply affected by the curse:

> The generational curse that we struggle with is not that birth is painful. In fact I don't even like calling it a curse. The only thing 'generational' we struggle with is our sin and the desire to blame others for what we experience. It is because of our sin we experience separation from God and we often focus on ourselves and not on God's purposes or plan. Just as sin is a generational sin, for women having multiplied pains in birth is generational. But our sin wants to call pain a curse or a burden… When we focus on the 'why' behind the pain, and face it with God's help rather than avoid it, then we can understand the greater purposes behind the pain, and see its worth.[3]

The problem with the view expressed in the above quote is that it avoids the fact the Bible expressly says that multiplied pain in childbearing is a result of the curse. The Bible uses the pain of childbirth as imagery for terrible and unavoidable suffering. It is not sinful to call pain a curse or a burden; it is true. To name this is to appropriately grieve over sin and seek redemption in the One who can set us free. The 'why' behind the pain is not the blessing of a child. The 'why' behind the pain is the devastation of sin. Beauty is not ultimately found in embracing this and letting it be, but rather in seeking freedom from its pervasive devastation and suffering through the death and resurrection of Jesus.

To brush over the fact of suffering in birth as though the process is not essentially marred, is also to diminish the goodness of God's original design. Childbirth is not being experienced as the perfectly beautiful and good thing it was first created to be. When we act as though it is even close to this, we lower the standard of God's goodness in his creation. We need to understand this in two equally important truths: On the one hand, childbirth was created by God, and it is good to bear children. On the other, because of the curse our sin evoked, it now involves pain and suffering that it was never originally intended to have. This means children are brought into the world at great personal cost to the mother. This teaches us something important about God, and about the world and redemption. We will miss the depth and beauty of this gospel understanding if we do not accept what sin has done to this process.

The availability of modern medical care and intervention, including pain relief, can be received as a blessing and means of grace. These medical interventions assist women in giving birth more comfortably and with less trauma than they would otherwise. The reality is that they save millions of lives. This should be seen as a blessing, and not something to be condemned or avoided, as though it works against God's design. In reality it can be a means of grace that saves us from some of the consequences of original sin.

It can also be true that this same modern interventional approach to childbirth may sometimes cause more harm than good. Some women who could give birth without intervention, feel pressured into unnecessary intervention during birth, and this can be damaging to either the mother or child. In many cases there is a mistrust of the natural process of childbirth, as though giving birth is something that women ideally need to do with medical assistance. There is good reason to question this viewpoint as natural childbirth is both possible and healthy in many Western contexts.

On the other hand, there are many times where medical intervention is needed, and the availability of such care means that childbirth is a much safer process than it has been in the past. These interventions are available to be used gladly and wisely, and without shame.

A philosophy that pushes the ideal of natural birth to the exclusion of all else often causes women to feel shame, failure or guilt, and is not only unchristian but also naive. It can only exist in the West, with our ready access to medical care. Natural birth ideals exist because of medical backup; natural birth without these backups can result in many women and babies dying. People in primitive conditions have no ideals surrounding childbirth; they understand its inevitable suffering and the real possibility of death.

Natural childbirth proponents tend to underestimate (or be totally ignorant of) how badly sin has affected childbearing, while the medical view can overlook the functionality of what still remains of God's good design.

I believe there is a third way, one in which we can acknowledge the goodness of God's design in the blessings of children whilst still facing the reality of the consequences of sin. In doing so we will find that redemption is most often found not in avoiding or minimising pain, but on the other side of it. This points us to Jesus, who endured the pain and shame of the cross. It is in *him* and his willingness to suffer that we find childbearing redeemed.

CHAPTER NINE

You Are Not Alone

Yea, in the night, my Soul, my daughter,
Cry – clinging to Heaven by the hems;
And lo, Christ walking on the water,
Not of Genesareth, but Thames!

– Francis Thompson [4]

There was a time that I believed that Jesus was uninvolved with the feminine pain of childbearing. I *wanted* to believe that Jesus sympathised with my weakness, but it was hard to imagine how he could. He had never been a woman, and had never been pregnant, so it seemed unrealistic for the writer of Hebrews to say that he has been tempted in every way we are (Hebrews 4:15-16).[5] I didn't want general sympathy for humanity, I wanted a Jesus who lived *my* humanity, who experienced the temptations peculiar to womanhood.

During my journaling and painful seeking I revisited basic questions such as 'What is womanhood?' I wanted to know how it was that God, who is 'Father' and sent us his 'Son', could truly walk in my childbirth shoes. Just as in *The Sound of Music* Julie

Andrews taught the Von Trapp children, 'Let's start at the very beginning, a very good place to start', I went back to the beginning, to the creation story.

> Then God said, 'Let us make man in our image, after our likeness. And let them have dominion over the fish of the sea and over the birds of the heavens and over the livestock and over all the earth and over every creeping thing that creeps on the earth.' So God created man in his own image, in the image of God he created him; male and female he created them. (Genesis 1:26-27)

This text represented the first obstacle I needed help to overcome. When God spoke about making man in his image, what did he mean? Is he just talking about males? If he was, I would have found no help. But the word 'man' refers to mankind in general, something which is more clearly expressed, where God speaks of 'them', and as being 'male and female'. The powerful news here is that God made both men and women in his image, after his likeness. As a woman I too reflect his image.

Femininity and womanhood say something about God. Jesus incarnate is male, but although God is always spoken about in a masculine context, he is not male or female; he is God. He is not human, and yet the fullness of humanity, man and woman, bear the likeness and image of God.

But how does Jesus know what it is like to be a woman in this context? How *can* he know?

He knows not only because he is God, but also because he became human. Beyond being men and women, we are human beings – mankind. And God entered into this humanity in the person of Jesus.

Jesus experienced birth in the same way every person experiences it; he was born just like us all. Through childbirth – messy, bloody, intimate and intensely human – he entered the world.

Jesus was 'a man of sorrows and acquainted with grief' (Isaiah 53). He suffered because of sin. It was not through his own personal sin, or moral failing to keep God's law – he fulfilled the law perfectly – but because he lived his life in the context of a sinful, broken world. And he, like us, experienced sorrow and distress because of this.

It is helpful to understand these things so that when you suffer in childbearing, you will be aware that this is the consequence of living in a world corrupted and broken by sin rather than your own personal moral failing against God.

'This is not good!' we cry out to God as we hang over the toilet day after day, or as we lie bedridden or unwell, our body groaning. And we are right. This is not his perfect creation; we are far from Eden. It is not wrong to bewail the pain of childbearing; it is sane. Jesus did not walk the earth endlessly praising God's good creation. He knew what a very good creation looked like, and how far we had fallen from that. He was grieved and sorrowed by what he experienced.

Jesus knew what life was like in Eden; he *created* it and he walked in it. He watched it become futile and fractured. If we think we experience pain in a broken world, we must realise that Jesus, knowing the glory of his original creation, must have felt this pain infinitely more intensely than we ever will.

In his pain Jesus moved towards the cross. Knowing that this was why he came, he prayed in the Garden of Gethsemane that there might be another way. He knew there wasn't. Deep sorrow and grief filled his soul. This was no smiling Saviour, going calmly on his way to save the world, knowing his pain had a purpose. This was a person who knew the depth of the suffering he was about to endure, and felt it to be unbearable. This was someone who knew our humanity – the willingness of the spirit and the weakness of the flesh shrinking from pain and death.

Jesus knew that this suffering was the will of his Father and would bring both joy and glory to himself. He wanted to give life and light to his children who were perishing in darkness and sin because of his great love for them. He knew this was the only way. He was willing. But he was in profound agony, and sweat like blood dripped from his body, even as an angel from heaven strengthened him.

During my second labour sweat dripped off my body. It dampened my hair and dripped off the straggling ends. I was in agony which I could not escape from. Pain seared through my body. My husband and the midwives supported me, but they could not ease the torturous pain. They fanned me with a giant palm leaf fan, but the sweat continued to pour. Even then, whilst sweating in agony, I knew that I was not alone. Jesus knew what I was going through and, hard as it is to even imagine, his agony was deeper and fuller than mine could ever have been!

Jesus, despite praying that he be spared, was crucified. He suffered unthinkable physical pain and took the curse on himself (Galatians 3:13).[6] If we had imagined he does not understand what it is to bear the curse of Genesis 3:16 in our body, we are quite mistaken. He carried the full weight of it in his body as he hung on the cross. He understands more fully than I ever will, the depth of that curse and its far-reaching effects. Here we finally see the woman's offspring bruising the serpent's head. Children are a blessing: here is the Blessed One setting humanity and creation free.

I entitled this chapter 'Not Alone', hoping to encourage and remind you that even in our most personal and vulnerable suffering as women in childbearing, we are not alone – Jesus has also known suffering. We can always see him right here with us, knowing us, loving us, intimately involved with us.

Jesus, however, knows something we will never know. While he hung on the cross and became a curse for us, his perfect, loving and intimate relationship with the Father was severed, and he experienced his Father's wrath and punishment for the sins of all humanity. When we find ourselves there at the cross with Jesus, tasting the bitterness of pain, agony and suffering, we must also see that Jesus drank the cup of God's wrath, a just fury that we will never taste. While we are not immune from the pain of a broken and cursed world, we find freedom in Christ. In our suffering we know the perfect love of our Father, even as we live and suffer imperfectly. As we repent of our sins and allow his Holy Spirit to live in us, we know his grace and his joy. In his suffering Jesus was cut off from the Father's perfect love, and instead experienced his Father's divine wrath and justice against sin. Because of this we are enabled to experience his grace and joy, as the penalty for sin has been paid.

Having had our sins atoned for, we may now live in complete freedom from the guilt and shame which entered the world with sin. Jesus suffered the shame of the cross, the guilt that we should have borne. In him we are without guilt and unashamed. How can we fully comprehend this freedom? It is perhaps so dazzling that we hide our eyes, more accustomed to the half-darkness of our sense of condemnation. We have freedom in Jesus to enter into light and life with him, where there is no condemnation. Shame is covered and guilt atoned for.

Our physical suffering then should not make us feel distant from Jesus, but rather intimately known by him. We are able to name our pain for what it is, not mask or hide it under platitudes about God's goodness. With the same sweat-stained lips that tremble in weakness and agony, we are able to praise Jesus for the pain we have been spared – the guilt and shame we have been freed from – and give thanks for the joy of his continual presence and perfect love.

Theologians refer to this willingness of Jesus to walk in our shoes and share in our sufferings as 'the sympathy of Christ':

> They [grief, friendship, fear] were the affections of an acutely sensitive human soul, alive to all the tenderness, and hopes, and anguish with which human life is filled… The present manhood of Christ conveys this deeply important truth, that the Divine heart is human in its sympathies.[7]

So far this is non-specific. We speak of anguish, sorrow and suffering. But in regard to childbearing, what kind of pains are we to seek Jesus' companionship in? To help answer this question, we can name specific ways we experience pain or suffering in childbearing. Some of them are intimate, and it may feel strange to think of Jesus being with you in this state of naked, raw suffering. But it is here that we need him most. We need not feel ashamed. He knows what it is to suffer the humiliation of naked pain. He doesn't flinch at ours.

Before we begin, I want you to know that it is not my intention to cause anxiety or fear. Rather, by naming what is often suffered silently and in the shadows, I hope that I can give voice to that pain, and lead you to find solace in the empathy of Christ.

Pains in childbearing are many and varied. It seems in *every* area related to reproduction there are common ways in which women experience suffering of one kind or another. I would like to mention some of these, in the hope that they will help us to think about people who have stories that are different (or perhaps similar) to our own. It is important to hear all of them.

There is more to childbearing than giving birth. Genesis 3 refers to more than merely the labour and delivery of a baby, although pain usually reaches its culmination and is most intensified at this point. Pain and suffering potentially span all of a woman's reproductive years.

Some suffer crippling pain each month with their period. Period pain or cramping is considered normal, but there are times when it is an indication that something about this process is not working as it should. One woman describes period pain whilst living with endometriosis:

> The pain is deep and heavy, almost as though I'm being pulled down by gravity. It's a soreness, sometimes a pinch or a twinge or even a stab – but nearly always it is just deep and full, almost like a moan that stays always in a low octave. There are times at night I find I can't move because it has pulled me down against my bed, where I find that I, too, must audibly groan, almost as though I'm harmonising with the depth of the painful chord inside.
>
> When it is tired and much heavier than usual, it will fall against my lower back. It sits there and pushes against my spine. I try not to tense, which only makes it worse, but even when I try to relax, or breathe, it makes little difference. The pain is not something I can guard against nor can I breathe into it – to breathe into it would be no less irritating than to fill a balloon to near bursting – and at times, that's exactly how it feels. Sometimes I realise I am

holding my breath and when I let it go, my legs shake and I feel a swell of pain that ripples through me as though it was a vibration from a hard-hit chord…

…People tell me just to relax. Doctors say it and well-meaning friends. Anyone who has ever borne witness to the pain implores me to relax. I no longer have control over this situation, you must understand. I can breathe in and around and within the pain – but that's the thing, I am in pain. I am living inside of it. That's what I'm saying when I say, 'I am in pain' – because to feel a pain so raw and deep and penetrating is to exist on a separate plane as each pulse moves through you, as though your internal organs are being bruised and beaten'.[8]

Premenstrual Syndrome (PMS), also known as PMT (Pre-menstrual Tension), can make life difficult for women each month. Many find that they easily become irritable and unreasonable. In extreme cases intense anger bottles up and becomes uncontrollable; a dark cloud covers everything; joy is sucked out of life and we regard the world with a sense of doom. This kind of stress (and in some cases oppression) each month can hinder a woman in her daily life and relationships, making ordinary problems feel heavier and sometimes overwhelming. We are robbed of joy, and lash out at those we love the most, even as we are trying to formulate a more godly response. Guilt and shame condemn us. Then it passes, only to return a few weeks later.

It may have been high school sex-education which first mentioned it, or maybe it was discussed in the school grounds, but it is commonly known that sex for girls is often painful the first time. In reality it can be painful for much longer than that. For a variety of reasons women may experience pain during sex on an ongoing basis. One newly-married Christian woman spent two years feeling like an inadequate wife because of her lack of desire as a consequence of terribly painful sex. Feeling that something was wrong with her, and having been made to understand before she got married that she must keep her husband happy or his 'eye would wander', she felt a deep sense of failure and shame.

For some women, sex has become dominated by the desire to conceive. There is a monthly cycle of hope, then grief and loss; hope against hope, and grief upon grief; an empty body and empty arms, all the while watching the arms of those around them gradually being filled. Grief, loss, anger, shame, bitterness and loneliness form the rhythm of their days. These women may ask the haunting question, 'Am I less of a woman if I cannot have children?' If we are tempted to think that motherhood fulfils God's purpose for women, we must revisit Eden before the fall. Eve had not yet conceived, carried a child or given birth, but she was, as God's creation, the perfect woman. God looked at all he had made, including Eve, and declared it 'very good'. God's purpose for women is not, ultimately, motherhood – it is to be like him. And this purpose is fulfilled in Christ. Let his eyes look at you long and deep, eyes filled with compassion for your loss and pain, eyes which give you dignity and worth as they delight in you. He looks at you with no condemnation – only grace and love. Jesus does not look and see a woman who lacks a child – he sees his child, precious, valued and complete in him.

There are women who will go through life without children of their own. These are women for whom childbearing never came, or at least never reached the point of delivering a living baby. They may have to deal with the guilt, shame, failure, loneliness and pain of never being a mother. One of these women put into words her own journey:

But still, it was hard. At first, the truth of my situation hit more and more deeply. Each time I thought: 'When I have a baby…' or 'My children will…' the pain hit anew. I wouldn't be having a baby. My children would never … and this got worse before it got better, like punching a bruise that is already tender.

But it did get better. Gradually I realised that punching the bruise was pointless, and so my brain trained itself not to think about the babies I didn't have, would never have. My brain stopped me thinking of myself as a mother. This took time. But the good minutes, then hours, then days, then weeks, came more frequently. At times I fought against it, feeling guilty that – on the good days – I was not grieving enough. I wondered, if I didn't continue to grieve and mourn the life I thought I would have, then maybe that meant I didn't really ever want it, or if it meant I was upset simply because I didn't get what I thought I wanted. So I wondered if my pain was fake, wondering if I didn't really have permission to feel pain, if it meant I, in fact, deserved what had happened. Of course, now I look back and know my grief and pain were legitimate. But still, the process of recovery itself made me feel guilty.

But healing is a gradual process, and so gradually I realised that this endless sadness would not serve me well. Back in the early days, immediately after my ectopic losses, I had felt the power of joy, even with something as simple as a joke on a sitcom, or the warmth of the sun on my back, a favourite song, or sitting looking out at the sea and a blue sky. Grasping joy as it came, even when it was fleeting, was what healed me.[9]

Conception does not always lead to having a healthy baby in your arms. Miscarriage is common in the first twelve weeks of pregnancy, but it being common does not make it any less of a loss. To the rest of the world your child was a vague reality, or perhaps they never even knew of it. But as a mother-to-be, your child lived. There was a due date for their birth, and you imagined them having a life, a future, a name and a personality. You loved and cherished a life that would never come into the world. Your grief and loss is not just for the unborn child, but for the child who will never be born.

Many women will attend their scans, hear the results of tests, and feel the weight of the curse bearing down on them afresh. Something is wrong – the baby will need surgery; the child will be disabled; the newborn will not survive. The world has suddenly become broken and imperfect, and now this is no longer a distant, impersonal theological doctrine. The reality of this broken imperfection, devastating and relentless, invades your life. You hold this brokenness in your body. You grieve for the loss of a healthy child, the child you expected and planned for, and for the life you wanted to give that child. You are unable to avoid the suffering, or to take away the sentence of suffering from your child. You may rage in grief-stricken pain. You may question that God is still good. But you will never again need to question the existence of suffering and pain.

Throughout pregnancy there are many discomforts and ills. There are ones that are merely annoying, and there are those which are debilitating. 'Morning sickness' must have been named by a male who had never experienced it. It is not limited to the morning, but is experienced all day, every day. Sometimes there are things which will help, but in many cases nothing will stop the relentless nausea and vomiting. Insomnia can drive you to the brink of insanity. Some women experience depression in pregnancy. For them pregnancy is not a time when you bloom, it is not precious or wonderful. Rather it means banishment to a world which is drained of colour, where hope is lost and joy is not found. As their baby grows within them, so does the darkness, hopelessness and fear. People are happy for them, and yet they have become numb to happiness and embittered toward life. They strive for control over their mind and emotions, but to no avail. They may more easily relate to the demon-possessed man who raved alone among the tombs than to Elizabeth or Mary who sang songs of praise to God for the babies they carried within them (Mark 5:1-20; Luke 1:39-56). But there is good news for those of us losing our minds on the outskirts of society – Jesus has arrived. He walks among the tombs and he heals the oppressed.

Birth is painful, but in the Western World we live under the illusion that it is not really dangerous, and we do not imagine that we could die, or that our baby could not survive. The reality is that even with all the access to medical care we have, some women will die. Babies are sometimes stillborn. Painful labour, anguish and death are still real possibilities.

Losing a baby in this way is cruel, ugly and relentless. I cannot imagine the sorrow of labouring, only to deliver a baby who has no life left in it. I think of Jesus weeping at the tomb of Lazarus, weeping with those who had lost someone they loved, deeply moved and troubled as he sees their sorrow. This is not how it is supposed to be. And Jesus wept (John 11:28-44).

Pregnancy can feel like the never-ending story, but for some the story ends too soon. Premature babies face extra, life-threatening challenges. One mother described her experience like this:

My first pregnancy and childbirth were not at all how I expected. My waters broke at 26 weeks and my son was born at 29+5. Every day after my waters broke was a bittersweet mix of disappointment, anxiety and guilt combined with joy and relief that our baby was still doing okay. In hindsight the birth was quite terrible. I suspect the pain was worsened by the lack of waters and because it was my first I had no idea of how much worse it might get and how much longer it would be. No epidural, just gas. I didn't feel in control of the situation, I was led entirely by the flock of medical staff on what to do and when. I didn't feel distinct contractions when I was being told to push and I suspect the midwife was pressing down to stimulate contracting when mine weren't coming fast enough to get baby out. It hurt. I was left feeling bruised and scarred by the whole experience but mostly I blocked it out as I was too busy afterwards with our little premature baby and a whole new world of concerns.

The stress of dealing with these situations can lead to other manifestations of post-natal distress. These include post-natal depression, where the burden of depression is coupled with the burden of caring for a newborn baby. Others experience post-traumatic stress disorder (PTSD), or post-partum psychosis. Sleep deprivation tortures most new mothers. All of these things can be devastating for those involved. Mothers who struggle with these post-partum disorders often feel their suffering compounded by guilt and shame. They may be unable to care for their child for a time, or struggle to feel a bond with them. Their babies may have to be cared for by family members or even strangers, while they are forced to take medication and are enclosed in the walls of a mental health ward.

Birthdays can become difficult reminders of a time they would rather forget. Love for the child can be slow in coming. The following is an excerpt from my journal:

> Today is my son's fourth birthday, and I have been thinking about how much has changed since that day he was born.
>
> I have realised it is not all over. I don't know if it ever will be. I have learned there is a name for this – post-natal PTSD. Looking back, I can see that each year my anxiety and stress around my son's birthday manifests in different ways. The first year it was obvious. I dreaded it. It was hard to celebrate his 'birth day'. I phrased the party invitation carefully, so as to celebrate his life rather than his birth. Numbness had become the norm since his birth, as well as underlying guilt and desperation. But we had a party, ate cake, wore party hats and sang 'Happy Birthday'. My stomach was tied in knots as I thought about 'this time last year…' Relief flooded over me when I realised that he had been born shortly after midnight, and that the anniversary of that moment had passed while I slept.
>
> The second year there were the tiredness and symptoms I usually feel when I am pregnant – migraines, inability to sleep and depression. Convinced I was pregnant, I did a pregnancy test. It was negative.
>
> The third year, in the midst of the new-baby madness, I recorded in my journal on the day before his birthday a feeling of uncertainty, fear and anxiety hovering over me.

I felt a sense of oppression. I didn't know what it was. I do now.

But getting help, and understanding what is going on, has given me hope that although this might never entirely be over, it will not continue to overwhelm me. This has been a hard week – I have had trouble sleeping, had bad headaches, and have been very tired. Yesterday by the time his party started I felt like hiding in bed. But I knew the reason for all of this, and that it was okay and would pass. I have made much progress since I first reached out for help that day in my doctor's office, when I told her, through painful, broken tears, the story of his birth. I can speak of it now without crying. I can hear others talk of giving birth without an anxiety attack. I can see a pregnant woman these days, without being overcome by feelings of revulsion.

I've even been pregnant again. I've had another child, and faced my worst fears in doing so. It has resulted in there being one more date on the calendar which haunts me each year. But it has also given me a baby who brought me more joy than I could ever have imagined.

There are women who will not be able to have children as a result of sexual abuse. There are survivors of sexual abuse who will suffer flashbacks and be re-traumatised during the birth process. Listen to this account from one such woman:

> Before I got pregnant, it never occurred to me that labour and childbirth could re-trigger sexual trauma for me in such significant ways. As a survivor of sexual violence, I

had more than twenty years of healing and recovery under my belt. But I was still completely unprepared for the ways in which birth – and the silence around it – would open so many old wounds in new ways.

Overall, pregnancy, labour and delivery were unlike any other experiences I had in my body or in my life. The energy I usually had available to manage my anxieties and emotions was being used in other ways, leaving me less resilient to new trauma. It required me to face new sensations that were scary and uncomfortable. On the one hand, it's an amazing experience to create life and to feel your heart open to a new human. On the other hand, many of the sensations were at the 'scene of the crime,' which left me feeling like a survivor.[10]

Even women who felt as though their births went well, and who gave birth naturally, may use the language of pain to describe their experience. Here are some of their own words:

I thought, 'There is no way I can move, I'm so tired.' But then I'd feel my body doing exactly what they asked.

I remember thinking that I was going to die, that really no baby was worth this pain and that actually I didn't want kids after all…

I was experiencing such intense, horrible pain… I was TERRIFIED of giving birth again. I remembered that last time the pain had been worse than I thought possible. I had forgotten how painful and awful that feeling of your body splitting in half is… I was still in shock and couldn't stop shaking for quite a while after she was born.

It was so hard to get my head back in the right space then. Part of me was ready to give up and go to hospital for an epidural.

The contractions were so painful at this point, I didn't know if I could continue.

Not many births in the Bible are described with any detail. Most often the women mentioned simply 'bore' or 'gave birth to' a son or daughter. But occasionally we are given a fuller story. There are three women that come to mind, whose childbirth experiences we hear something about: Rebekah, Tamar and the unnamed wife of Phinehas.

In Genesis 25:19-27 we read about Rebekah. Rebekah was infertile, but her husband prayed and God granted his prayer – and she became pregnant with twins. For someone who had wanted this more than anything in the world, it must have been a difficult and disappointing time to have a pregnancy so bad that she found herself saying, 'If it's going to be this bad, why am I even alive?' (Genesis 25:22)[11] When they were born, the first one came out covered in red hair. The second came out hand first, holding his brother's heel. This is all recorded matter-of-factly, but if we stop to think for a moment about a birth where a baby arrives hand first, attached to his brother, we will realise how difficult it must have been for Rebekah. I would venture to say that this was a difficult birth.

Genesis 28 tells the tragic story of Tamar. Tamar, the widow of an evil man, was sexually misused by her brother-in-law and impregnated by her father-in-law, who thought she was a prostitute. Subsequently she laboured to give birth to twins. The first baby descended, hand first. In what must have been an agonising delivery, before he was delivered he retreated and the other twin was born first. Even the midwife was moved to exclaim about this complicated breach birth.

In 1 Samuel 4:19-22 we read the story of an unnamed woman who was the wife of Phinehas and therefore the daughter-in-law of the prophet Samuel. She went into labour after hearing the devastating news that her husband and father-in-law had both been killed in battle, and that the Ark of the Covenant had been captured. She gave birth to a son, but lacked the will to go on living after the news of such devastating loss. The midwife tried to rally her with the good news of a baby boy, but she did not respond before she passed away.

As we read the birth stories the Bible gives us, it ceases to surprise us that when the Bible speaks of childbirth, it uses words such as 'anguish', 'dismay', 'writhing', 'pangs', 'groaning', 'crying out' and 'sorrow'.

Childbearing also will take its toll on a woman's body. There are varying degrees of damage. Some of us will merely live with some stretch marks, saggy breasts and loose skin around the belly. But there are many other ways our body may be affected. Rips and tears from deliveries need stitches. Prolapses occurs. Bladder weakness becomes part of life. Stomach muscles separate, and the damage caused by a caesarean section may leave the body scarred and disfigured.

One woman, after an extensive emergency caesarean to deliver her 11lb baby, was left with large flaps of scarred skin, even after she lost the 45kg she had put on during pregnancy.

Unable to wear many normal items of clothing because of the extra skin, she looked to surgery to get it removed. She has experienced judgement from other Christian women for doing so, as though deformities caused by childbirth are somehow sacred, and the desire to fix them is worldly and a rejection of God's gift of motherhood.

Yet there is another body which bears the scars that speak of new life bought at a cost. With holes in his hands, feet and side, Jesus invites us to view the reality of sin-scarred flesh. But he also offers healing. By God's gracious provision of medical and surgical intervention, our bodies can seek healing from the things which went wrong as we gave birth. We are right to think some scars are sacred, but *these* ones are not ours, they are Christ's.

It's not just mothers who endure a form of agony as they give birth; the loving husbands standing by also feel the pain of helplessness as they witness such anguish. One man, his children now adults, recalls how he felt as he witnessed the birth of his children:

> It took me a while to like my kids, let alone love them. I just felt bad for the terrible time my wife had had. As a bystander, it's a horrible thing to witness.

Then, at the end of the childbearing years, our bodies and emotions often suffer again during the time of menopause. Hot flushes, mood changes, lack of interest in sex, painful sex and other physical and emotional symptoms may be experienced. So we see that from the beginning to the end of our childbearing years, there are many ways in which we are plagued by pain and suffering.

It is important to hear these stories. They may make us

uncomfortable and not fit well with our ideology. But if we are going to find a purpose in the pain and redemption from this broken process, we must take time to listen to the stories of women who have walked the road of suffering and who speak the language of pain.

A common thread in these stories of pain are the feelings of guilt and shame: What do we do with them? How do we find hope and freedom?

We come to Jesus. And as we listen we learn that he too speaks the language of pain.

CHAPTER TEN

Joy

O Joy that seekest me through pain,
I cannot close my heart to thee;
I trace the rainbow through the rain,
And feel the promise is not vain,
That morn shall tearless be.

– George Matheson [12]

With the advent of Jesus in the Biblical narrative, the imagery of childbearing changes. Before Jesus it was only negative. Mostly found in the Prophets, the imagery of childbirth was used to convey unavoidable pain and inevitable suffering. It is only referred to in these terms. But although Jesus also uses this language, something new is added to the imagery – joy.

If the pain of childbearing reminds us of the dreadful consequences of original sin – which in Christ has no ultimate power over us, though we feel its pangs – then it is only in the person of Christ that we discover the true meaning of childbirth. With the advent of Jesus, the Bible unfolds this metaphor for us further, and reveals that childbirth is a picture of suffering that leads to greater joy because of a new life given.

It is Jesus himself who first uses this imagery. In the gospel of John, he speaks to his disciples before he goes to the cross, encouraging and preparing them for the events which are about to happen:

> When a woman is giving birth, she has sorrow because her hour has come, but when she has delivered the baby, she no longer remembers the anguish, for joy that a human being has been born into the world. (John 16:21)

Here he speaks matter-of-factly about a woman's sorrow and anguish at the time of birth. Even though he is speaking here to his disciples, who are all men, this 'take' on childbirth is no surprise to them for they understand that childbirth brings sorrow and anguish. The imagery is accepted without question or explanation. But then Jesus speaks of something greater, something which surpasses the anguish, so that she 'no longer remembers' it. This is joy.

Jesus is mentoring his disciples and preparing them for what they are about to experience: great sorrow and loss, and then great joy in new life. In the light of Jesus' victory over sin and our subsequent freedom from the curse, childbearing takes on a new meaning. Now we see a fuller picture of what childbearing points us to. In Romans it is used as imagery again, not only as terrible and unavoidable suffering and judgement, but of pain endured in the hope of greater joy.

> For the creation was subjected to futility, not willingly, but because of him who subjected it, in hope that the creation

itself will be set free from its bondage to corruption and obtain the freedom of the glory of the children of God.

For we know that the whole creation has been groaning together in the pains of childbirth until now.

And not only the creation, but we ourselves, who have the first fruits of the Spirit, groan inwardly as we wait eagerly for adoption as sons, the redemption of our bodies. (Romans 8:20-23)

Later in Galatians, Paul also uses this imagery of childbirth, to express his enduring great pain in the hope of 'birthing' something far greater – God's redemptive work.

...my little children, for whom I am again in the anguish of childbirth until Christ is formed in you! (Galatians 4:19)

We begin now to see that childbearing is about more than a woman's ability to have children; it is about more than God's blessing of continued life for humanity; it speaks powerfully of sin and Jesus' victory over it, and of his willingness to suffer because of his great love and his deep joy in the salvation of his people. We see shadows of this in the Old Testament as it speaks of him:

Out of the anguish of his soul he shall see and be satisfied... (Isaiah 53:11)

Through childbearing women have a unique insight into this willingness to suffer because of hope of a greater joy. We know our health will suffer; our bodies will groan and falter under the burden. We know pain is coming, but we willingly walk this path for the joy set before us. When all is said and done, we look at our child with love in our eyes and say, 'It was worth it!'

After the birth of my first child, my joy and delight in her was so overwhelming that despite the fact that pregnancy had been filled with months of sickness, insomnia, backache and depression, I longed to have another baby and experience this joy again. I was willing to walk into months of suffering, culminating in the worst pain I had ever endured, because the joy at the end of it was so much greater than the suffering.

This theme of joy is important because it tells us not only about our own personal experience but also about God and his attitude towards the humanity he created in his image, even though we turned so terribly against him. It tells us something about how he relates to human beings, whom he allowed to live and suffer under the conditions recorded in chapter three of the book of Genesis.

Childbirth was always a theme of hope: one day a Saviour would be born. Yet it was also a brutal and sorrowful reminder of the conditions under which we live, and of the great need for redemption from them. Although childbirth is a symbol of hope and continued life for humanity, women and children would die in the process. Futility, corruption and decay characterise the world into which children are born. Violence, sickness, suffering and death are part of this world too.

But this was not God's final word on creation and humanity. *Jesus was coming*. He was coming to suffer under the conditions of this broken and cursed creation. He would suffer the full weight of sin, because of his great love for us.

Why was Jesus willing to suffer on our behalf? What motivated him to bear our guilt and shame? It was future joy. We read in the book of Hebrews:

Jesus, the founder and perfecter of our faith, who for the joy that was set before him endured the cross, despising the shame, and is seated at the right hand of the throne of God. (Hebrews 12:2)

Because of the joy set before him, Jesus went to the cross. He would see beyond the anguish of his soul, and be satisfied.

The moment of delivery for a woman in childbirth is most often one of relief and great joy, and overwhelming love. When Jesus says she will forget her anguish, he does not mean that she will develop sudden amnesia about the labour. Instead the word 'remember' conveys an active calling to mind. She forgets in the sense that she no longer calls to mind the pain, because of the greater joy in her child.

Zephaniah tells us the following:

The LORD your God is in your midst, a mighty one who will save; he will rejoice over you with gladness; he will quiet you by his love; he will exult over you with loud singing. (Zephaniah 3:17)

How many mothers have rejoiced over their children with gladness, quieted them with their love, and sung over them with a heart of exultation? How does God feel towards his children? He delights in them (Isaiah 62:4). He rejoices over them (Isaiah 62:5).

As we give our bodies and hearts and minds over to the task of bearing children, do we remember that God takes delight in us? Do we see him look at us with such great love and satisfaction that we *know* he thinks it is all worth it? Jesus delights in you.

But we have to remember that childbearing is an imperfect

image of this delight, as all human analogies of the Divine are. It does not always end in joy and new life. Many mothers have given birth to babies who have no life in them, and many mothers have lost their lives in the very process of *giving* it.

What can we say about joy when a mother's arms are left empty, or a baby cries with no mother to comfort it? Because of Jesus we can *still* speak of joy – a joy that does not leap up inside us like a songbird soaring in the summer sky, but rather as the solid ground beneath our feet when the light has drained out of the world, the pit engulfs us, and we can no longer see our way forward. In these times we cannot see joy, but only feel its presence under us, pressing against the weight of our body, not allowing us to fall any further, and enabling us to take another breath and carry on. It becomes a deep and steady chord that plays through even the saddest lament. It is more persistent than pain, and will outlast suffering. It is Jesus.

> He will wipe away every tear from their eyes, and death shall be no more, neither shall there be mourning, nor crying, nor pain anymore… (Revelation 21:4)

Epilogue

The theme of redemption ran through my third pregnancy like a scarlet thread, bright against the darkness that encompassed me, a guide that gave me hope. I thought of redemption as being in control and finishing strong with joy and peace. I didn't end that way. I ended broken and in anguish.

But I ended with Christ. I ended at the cross. And as I traced the theme of childbirth throughout the Bible, I understood that this is exactly where redemption is found. It was never about my personal strength and victory; it is about Jesus' ultimate victory over sin. Childbirth is redeemed in Christ as a symbol of the great redemption of all creation. New life. Joy. Peace. All these are found in Christ alone, through his suffering, death and resurrection.

Childbirth was redeemed, not because I didn't suffer, but because through it I came to see the glory of Christ suffering with me and on my behalf. I shared in his suffering, and I share in his victory. There was a depth of intimacy reached that could not have been reached had I not seen him with me through the blood, sweat and tears. When I couldn't go on, and the bitterness of failure tasted like death on my lips, I heard his voice as he carried me safely to the end:

Don't be afraid, for I have redeemed you. I am God, your Saviour. You are precious in my eyes, and honoured, and I love you. You are mine.[13]

Endnotes

1. Elizabeth Goudge, *The Scent of Water*, Hodder and Stoughton, 1963, p91.
2. Eugene Peterson, *Christ Plays in Ten Thousand Places*, Hodder & Stoughton 2005, p58.
3. Angie Tolpin, *Redeeming Childbirth: Experiencing His Presence in Pregnancy, Labor, Childbirth, and Beyond*, Crossbooks, 2013, p143.
4. Francis Thompson, 'The Kingdom of God'.
5. Hebrews 4:15-16, 'For we do not have a high priest who is unable to sympathise with our weaknesses, but one who in every respect has been tempted as we are, yet without sin. Let us then with confidence draw near to the throne of grace, that we may receive mercy and find grace to help in time of need.'
6. Galatians 3:13, 'Christ redeemed us from the curse of the law by becoming a curse for us'.
7. Robertson, Frederick W, 'Sermon 7: The Sympathy of Christ', www.fwrobertson.com/sermons/ser07.htm, Accessed 08/08/16.
8. Abbie Norman, 'This is what endometriosis feels like',

www.huffingtonpost.com/abby-norman/this-is-what-endometriosi_b_5704273.html, Accessed 19/5/15.
9. nokiddinginnz.blogspot.co.nz/p/my-story.html, Accessed 19/5/15.
10. Sarah Beaulieu, 'A Sexual Assault Survivor's Reflections on Birth', www.huffingtonpost.com/sarah-beaulieu/a-sexual-assault-survivors-reflections-on-birth_b_4831780.html, Accessed 8/10/15.
11. Genesis 25:22, 'If it is thus, why is this happening to me?'
12. George Matheson, 'O love that wilt not let me go'.
13. Isaiah 43:1-4, 'But now thus says the Lord, he who created you, O Jacob, he who formed you, O Israel: "Fear not, for I have redeemed you; I have called you by name, you are mine. When you pass through the waters, I will be with you; and through the rivers, they shall not overwhelm you; when you walk through fire you shall not be burned, and the flame shall not consume you. For I am the Lord your God, the Holy One of Israel, your Saviour. I give Egypt as your ransom, Cush and Seba in exchange for you. Because you are precious in my eyes, and honoured, and I love you, I give men in return for you, peoples in exchange for your life."'

About the Author
(In the words of her children)

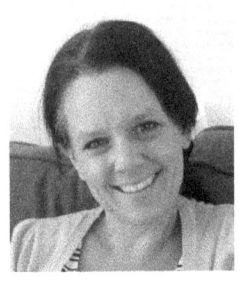

This is the truth, the only truth, about what Anna is like.

Anna Vroon lives in Gisborne, New Zealand, with her husband Bruwer and four kids. Three of them are boisterous boys but one of them is a beautiful young lady who isn't bossy, just gives advice. Anna deals with the noise better than most. I don't know how, that is one of the few things that remain a mystery.

Bruwer and Anna have fostered several extra babies and young children over the past five years. Anna enjoys writing, gardening, ballet and caring for babies (particularly the ones she doesn't have to birth herself).

She is keen on walking anywhere and everywhere. Sometimes she gets a bit angry. Sometimes she's really nice.

She is a lover of Christ our God and is an important member of Gisborne Grace Presbyterian Church where Bruwer is minister.

Sometimes she looks nice. She eats a lot. Sometimes she watches TV without us.

So there you have it. Anna Vroon: fun, (almost) faultless and completely surprising.

www.ingramcontent.com/pod-product-compliance
Lightning Source LLC
Chambersburg PA
CBHW051406290426
44108CB00015B/2173